Social aspects of illness, disease and sickness absence

Halvor Nordby, Rolf Rønning & Gunnar Tellnes (eds.)

Unipub 2011

© Unipub 2011

ISBN 978-82-7477-480-3

Contact info Unipub:
T: + 47 22 85 33 00
F: + 47 22 85 30 39
E-mail: post@unipub.no
www.unipub.no

Publisher: Oslo Academic Press, Unipub Norway
Printed in Norway: AIT Oslo AS

This book has been produced with economical support from
Østlandsforskning and Lillehammer University College.

All rights reserved. No part of this publication may be reproduced or
transmitted, in any form or by any means, without permission

Preface

In the summer of 2009 a Scandinavian research group from the *Social factors contributing to sickness absence* (*SOFAC*) project met in Sunne, Sweden, to discuss ongoing research concerning health problems and sickness absence. During these meetings, it became clear that we had a common interest in understanding social aspects of the processes leading to illness, disease and long-term sickness absence. The idea of a publication on this issue emerged, and this book – *Social aspects of illness, disease and sickness absence* – is the result.

Each chapter of the book examines the relational aspects of states of sickness – how they are influenced by social mechanisms and contextual factors. The idea is not merely that there is a strict causal connection between social relations and long-term sickness absence, but rather that the states of sickness have a dynamic and relational nature in themselves. Focusing on the individual incapacity for work without considering the psycho-social environment makes it impossible to understand some of the most important processes leading to long-term sickness absence. *Sickness absence* is, in this sense, a social concept – it applies to a phenomenon with an essentially interpersonal nature.

We hope that this book will become an indispensible resource for all those interested in understanding how long-term sickness absence can be conceived of as a dynamic and social phenomenon. First and foremost, the book aims to provide academics and researchers with an up-to-date analysis of long-term sickness absence and of relevant empirical research. The book can also be a valuable text for students in higher level courses that focus on the relation between individuals' health and their psycho-social environment.

In addition, those with a practical or public interest in long-term sickness absence may find the analyses that the book presents useful, in particular, for communicative purposes. Doctors and social workers can acquire valuable 'conceptual tools' for understanding absentees' life-worlds and the way they experience their own situation.

This book is a multidisciplinary publication with contributions from researchers working in Lillehammer University College, Eastern Norway Research Institute, University of Karlstad, Sweden, Gjøvik University College and Institute of Health and Society, University of Oslo. We want to thank the Norwegian Research Council for funding the SOFAC project, and Oslo Academic Press (Unipub) for publishing the book.

Oslo and Lillehammer October 1th, 2010
Halvor Nordby, Rolf Rønning and Gunnar Tellnes (editors)

Contents

Chapter 1
Research on long-term sickness absence:
The need for a wide methodological approach
Halvor Nordby, Rolf Rønning & Gunnar Tellnes 9

I. THEORETICAL PART

Chapter 2
On the concepts *disease*, *illness*, and *sickness*
Bjørn Hofmann 19

Chapter 3
On the dynamics of sickness in work absence
Bjørn Hofmann 47

Chapter 4
Sickness absence as a social construction: A theoretical perspective
Rolf Rønning 63

Chapter 5
Aspects of sickness certification and work ability
Gunnar Tellnes 83

Chapter 6
Disease, illness and long term sickness absence: A conceptual framework for categorising controversial cases
Halvor Nordby 93

Chapter 7
The subjectivity of illness, social roles and the harmful dysfunction analysis of disease
Halvor Nordby 111

Chapter 8
Social bonds, emotional processes and mental ill-health
Ulla-Britt Eriksson, Bengt Starrin,
Lena Ede & Staffan Janson 131

II. EMPIRICAL PART

Chapter 9
Influence of insecure social bonds at work and adverse life events: A comparison between long-term sickness absentees with mental diagnoses and a healthy population
Ulla-Britt Eriksson, Lars-Gunnar Engström,
Bengt Starrin & Staffan Janson 157

Chapter 10
The impact of psycho-social work environment on sickness absence: Results from the Swedish Life & Health 2008 Study
Lars-Gunnar Engström & Ulla-Britt Eriksson 175

Chapter 11
Working part-time for the sake of health
Lena Ede 185

Chapter 12
The benefits of nature and culture activities on health, environment and wellbeing: A presentation of three evaluation studies among persons with chronic illnesses and sickness absence in Norway
Kari Batt-Rawden & Gunnar Tellnes 199

Chapter 13
Helpers of the fragile, elderly and sick:
Report from a nursing home
Kari Batt-Rawden & Liv Johanne Solheim 223

Chapter 14
Absence and alternative learning: The Company Programme and inclusive working life as a means to reduce high school absence
Vegard Johansen, Tuva Schanke & Liv Johanne Solheim 243

Chapter 15
Social factors and long-term sickness absence: The need for a broader approach
Vegard Johansen & Rolf Rønning..265

Authors..285

Chapter 1

Research on long-term sickness absence: The need for a wide methodological approach

Halvor Nordby, Rolf Rønning & Gunnar Tellnes

Sickness absence can be studied in many ways from different practical and theoretical perspectives. This book will not attempt to argue that some of these perspectives are more fruitful or 'better' than the others. We do believe, however, that a satisfactory overall understanding of sickness absence, and of long-term sickness absence in particular, presupposes that two crucial conditions are met. The first condition is a requirement about methodology:

> (1) In order to shed light on some of the most important processes leading to sickness absence, empirical studies need to be combined with theoretical perspectives.

Obviously, quantitative and qualitative methods are fundamental to our scientific and practical knowledge of sickness absence. Empirical research can help us to understand why so many people are absent from work for longer periods due to health problems, and it can help us to prevent long-term sickness absence. But empirical investigations are not sufficient for the purpose of achieving a more *critical* understanding of the causes of long-term sickness absence. In our modern world, why are so many people suffering from mild mental disorders and 'modern' lifestyle illnesses like burnout? What can be done to reduce long-term sickness absence that is not caused by traditional somatic or severe psychological disorders?

It is imperative to go beneath numbers and directly observable data in order to arrive at sound answers to these questions. To understand and possibly reduce long-term sickness absence, it is necessary to adopt a *phenomenological* perspective that can help to clarify how absentees think about themselves and their life situations. It is also necessary to critically discuss the fundamental concepts that we use to describe the phenomena we are interested in. What is the conceptual relation between concepts like experienced *illness,* diagnosed *disease,* and the social role *sickness absence*? Is sickness absence always a negative concept – a concept that absentees experience as a problematic label? Or is it the case that some think of their status of being certified sick as a positive entitlement, a categorization that makes it easier for them to realise personal goals and achieve a fundamental 'sense of coherence'. These questions have dimensions that transcend the limitations of quantitative research and traditional empirical investigations.

Consequently, this book is divided into two parts. The first part presents theoretical explorations of the concept of *sickness absence* and related concepts like *illness* and *disease*. The main aim here is to give the reader a fundamental understanding of these and other basic concepts in the area. Some of the analyses have a further normative aim. They purport to clarify how the concepts should be understood. Many of the chapters use meta-analysis as an argumentative strategy. Conclusions about the status of our current knowledge and disputed concepts are based on discussions of existing empirical research.

In a multidisiplinary publication like this, there are quite often different traditions of concepts describing the same or similar phenomena. Some chapters (2, 3 and 6) present and discuss the subtle differences among these concepts, but in other chapters and the literature referenced, these concepts may be used interchangeably (e.g. sickness absence, sick leave, absenteeism, sick listing, sickness certification). Similarly, some authors may use different concepts to explain health problems, e.g. illness, disease, ill health, sickness, etc. In spite of this diverse use of terminology, we think that the reader will understand the conceptual references, i.e. the common meaning, of these words.

The second part of the book is empirical in a more traditional sense. The chapters in this part present empirical research that can help us to understand the practical consequences in Norway and Sweden related to social institutions and health policies in the two countries.

From a medical point of view, this research concerns doctors' sickness certification practice, the potential for prevention, functional and work ability assessments, and occupational rehabilitation in the field of absence from work. From a political point of view, it is important to have an understanding of all the different factors that contribute to sickness absence and of the possible interplay among them. Even for politicians, the right cures depend on adequate diagnoses.

The second condition that we think is crucial for understanding sickness absence, can be formulated as follows:

(2) States of illness and disease leading to sickness absence are relational states. Sickness absence is a social phenomenon that should be studied from a wide perspective that takes absentees' psycho-social environments into account.

We believe that our combined theoretical-empirical methodological strategy can give us the tools that are needed to shed light on this social dimension. The strategy can, in particular, be used to understand the most important 'grey cases'. Grey cases are here understood as disputed or controversial cases – cases in which it is not entirely evident whether an absentee should be, or needs to be, away from work.

A typical example might be 'burnout'. As emphasized in several chapters below, cases of 'burnout' normally involve absentees who have experienced that they cannot cope with all the formal and informal duties and obligations that they feel are expected of them. A good question to ask is whether the overall burden can be reduced, or whether it is possible to influence absentees' 'sense of coherence' or beliefs about their own capabilities in a more positive direction. In various ways, the chapters focus on this and other grey cases and argue that they have important social elements.

It is important to remember that, from a critical perspective, the grey cases are the most important, in particular for empirical and normative categorization. Any discussion of sickness absence with normative ambitions should therefore be measured against the need to say something useful about the grey cases. The discussion should have some implications for how the disputed grey cases should be understood and categorized. Most fundamentally, we believe that the value of this book can be measured by this requirement. We believe, and we hope the reader will agree, that our combined theoretical-empirical approach and our focus on social mechanisms give us resources to analyze some of the most difficult categories in a fruitful way.

Overview of the chapters

Theoretical part

In chapter 2, 'On the Concepts of disease, illness and sickness', Bjørn Hofmann presents and clarifies the traditional and very influential distinctions between disease, illness and sickness. The idea is that disease represents the medical profession's perspective on health problems, illness, the subjective first-person perspective, and sickness, the social perspective. This understanding forms a platform on which many of the other chapters are based. Readers who are unacquainted with the triad disease, illness and sickness should therefore read chapter 2, before moving on to the other discussions.

Chapter 3, 'On the dynamics of sickness in work absence', also written by Bjørn Hofmann, discusses the concept of sickness in more detail. He shows that the concept has a dynamic, relational character, and that the social dimensions of the concept become particularly striking when we attempt to understand the holistic character of long-term sickness absence. The chapter ends by outlining some normative implications of the conceptual relations that Bjørn develops.

In chapter 4, 'Sickness absence as a social construction: A theoretical perspective', Rolf Rønning outlines a moderate social constructionist framework for the understanding of sickness absence. Within a social constructionist model, the expansion of diagnoses and the growth in sickness absence can be seen as mechanisms for social control, in which medicine has the important function of controlling deviance in modern societies. The chapter also sheds light on medicine and pharmaceutical firms as instigators of the growth in sickness absence.

Gunnar Tellnes, in chapter 5, 'Aspects of sickness certification and work ability', describes and comments on the findings and recommodations from studies and theories related to doctors' sickness certification practice, the potential for prevention, functional and work ability assessments, and occupational rehabilitation in the field of absence from work. The chapter ends by commenting on the current practice and policy of social security in Norway and on the challenges that may result in relation to work ability assessment.

In chapter 6, 'Disease, illness and long-term sickness absence: A conceptual framework for categorising controversial cases', Halvor Nordby uses the concepts disease, illness and sickness (as presented by Hofmann in chapter 2) in a critical analysis of long-term sickness absence. The aim is to clarify 'grey' cases of long-term sickness absence – cases in which it is not obvious whether an absentee should be, or needs to be, absent from work. The chapter argues that many of these 'grey' cases involve illness, but no typical somatic severe mental pathological disorder. In addition, there are other important categories, such as a disease without subjective feeling of illness and sickness without experienced illness or a disease. The chapter ends by outlining an overall classification of some of the most important grey cases.

Chapter 7, 'The subjectivity of illness, social roles and the harmful dysfunction analysis of disease', also written by Halvor Nordby, focuses more narrowly on the concept of disease. His starting point is the fact that many controversial cases of long-term sickness absence involve genuine first-person negative experiences that have not been traced to traditional disease states. But does this mean that they do not involve disease at all? The chapter argues that influential definitions of disease actually imply that experienced illness and sick roles can be sufficient for disease. This means, the chapter concludes, that the question of whether illness and sickness absence can be sufficient for disease is a deeply philosophical one.

In chapter 8, 'Social bonds, emotional processes and mental ill-health', Ulla-Britt Eriksson, Bengt Starrin, Lena Ede and Staffan Janson discuss how theories of emotions can be used to understand sickness absence. The authors describe how emotions, particularly shame, seem to play an important role. Even though our knowledge of the frequency of shaming in the workplace is limited, some studies show that it is rather common. Having been condescended seems to be strongly associated with long-term sickness absence with a mental diagnosis. Finally, the chapter presents the hypothesis of the Burnout staircase. It describes a step-wise process toward sickness absence due to burnout.

Empirical part

Chapter 9, 'Influence of insecure social bonds at work and adverse life events: A comparison between long-term sickness absentees with mental diagnoses and a healthy population', written by Ulla-Britt Eriksson, Lars-Gunnar

Engstrøm, Bengt Starrin and Staffan Janson, tests the hypothesis of 'the Burnout staircase' presented in chapter 8. This is done by examining the association between psychosocial factors and sickness absence, while adding conflicts and losses in private life into the hypothesis. The main conclusion is that the burnout staircase seems to be a suitable model for describing sickness absence processes with a mental diagnosis, and that weak social bonds in private life should be included in the model.

Ulla-Britt Eriksson and Lars-Gunnar Engstrøm, in chapter 10, 'The impact of psycho-social work environment on sickness absence: Results from the Swedish Life and Health 2008 Study', examine the psychosocial working conditions of men and women in relation to sickness absence, by means of Karasek-Theorell's job strain model. The study is conducted on a large Swedish sample. It suggests that the changing labour market is important for explaining the effects the psychosocial work environment has on sickness absence in almost all types of jobs and, furthermore, that there may be a decreasing number of 'healthy jobs' in the Swedish labour market

In chapter 11, 'Working part time for the sake of health', Lena Ede presents a study of part-time employment in care work in Sweden. It has been a widespread assumption in public and political discourse that workers wish to work full-time in order to secure a sufficient income. Contrary to this, Lena shows that many care workers choose to work part-time for the sake of their own health, as a personal strategy for avoiding mental and physical health problems that would otherwise lead to sickness absence. The chapter concludes that this finding should be an important consideration in practical, ideological, and theoretical discussions of the idea that full-time work is a realistic normative ideal.

In chapter 12, 'The benefits of nature-culture activities on health, environment and well-being', Kari Batt-Rawden and Gunnar Tellnes present results from three evaluation studies, which focus on how art, music, nature, and culture have a beneficial impact on health and well-being. The studies have investigated the potential of nature-cultural-health based activities in terms of their health-promoting properties. A major finding is that nature-culture experiences, including a salutogenic perspective, may help the participants to construct experienced life meaning, identify coping mechanisms and revitalize the energetic and resourceful parts of the self. This type of research studies could stimulate future health promotion and rehabilitation programs in interdisciplinary cooperation.

Chapter 13, 'Fragile elderly and sick helpers: Report from a nursing home', by Kari Batt-Rawden and Liv Johanne Solheim, presents results from a qualitative study at a nursing home. Health and social services have been one of the branches with the highest rate of sickness absence in the recent past. A major finding of Batt-Rawden and Solheim's study is that the work overload seems to be the dominant reason for sickness absence. However, for some of the employees, problems in the private sphere were crucial factors. Furthermore, the role of being certified as sick influenced the participants' identities and made them vulnerable to being stigmatized.

In chapter 14, 'Absence and alternative learning: The company programme and inclusive working life as a means to reduce high school absence', Vegard Johansen, Tuva Schanke and Liv Johanne Solheim examine the influence of a European entrepreneurship program (CP) on school absence and dropout rates. There is a strong correlation between dropping out of secondary school and a high rate of sickness absence in later employment. Even though we know about this correlation, there are few studies on school absence and young people's attitudes towards absence. This chapter contributes to filling the gap and concludes that programs like CP can reduce school absence.

In chapter 15, 'Social factors and long-term sickness absence: The need for a broader approach', Vegard Johansen and Rolf Rønning test the influence of social factors on long-term sickness absence, using data from a standard of living study conducted in two Norwegian municipalities. Differences in sickness absence rates are often explained by demographic factors, family relations, socio-economic status, and work-place characteristics. The data used in this study allows the authors to include indicators of social integration in society and of life-style. It is shown that daily smoking and obesity are correlated with a high level of sickness absence. The same is true for people rarely visited by others and those without friends to serve as confidants.

All the authors of the chapters of this book agree that sickness absence can be studied in many ways from different practical and theoretical perspectives. It is our hope that the book can help the readers to achieve a better understanding of the interdisiplinary and complex phenomenon of long-term sickness absence in the light of health problems like illness, disease, and injuries.

I. Theoretical part

Chapter 2

On the concepts *disease, illness,* and *sickness*

Bjørn Hofmann

Summary

The point of departure for this chapter is a review of the discussion between Andrew Twaddle and Lennart Nordenfelt on the concepts of disease, illness, and sickness. The objective is to investigate the fruitfulness of these concepts for modern health care. It is argued that disease, illness, and sickness represent different perspectives on human ailment and that they can be applied to analyse both epistemic and normative challenges to modern medicine. In particular, the analysis reveals epistemic and normative differences among the concepts. Furthermore, the discussion demonstrates, against Nordenfelt, that the concepts of disease, illness, and sickness can exist independently of a general theory of health. Additionally, the complexity of different perspectives on human ailment also explains why it is so difficult to give strict definitions of basic concepts within modern health care.

Introduction

The triad of *disease, illness,* and *sickness* has been applied to denote medical, personal, and social aspects of human ailment respectively.[1] The distinction

---

[1] *Ailment* here denotes negative bodily occurrence and is applied as a common term to refer to disease, illness, sickness, injury, defect, disability, handicap and impairment.

between illness and disease has been noted in theoretical medicine since the 1950's (Parsons 1951; 1958; 1964; Feinstein 1967). Andrew Twaddle first elaborated on the distinction between disease, illness, and sickness in his doctoral dissertation defended in 1967 (Twaddle 1968; Twaddle 1994a, 22). The distinctions between *disease, illness*, and *sickness* have become commonplace in medical sociology, medical anthropology, and philosophy of medicine.[2]

In recent years, the triad has been elaborated and more strictly defined (Sachs 1988; Twaddle 1994a; 1994b), but also fundamentally challenged (Nordenfelt 1994; Nordenfelt 2007). Lennart Nordenfelt has argued that the triad[3] is fruitful only within the context of a general theory of health (Nordenfelt 1987; 1994).

The point of departure for this chapter is the debate about the triad between Twaddle and Nordenfelt (Twaddle 1994a; 1994b; Nordenfelt 1994). Its objective is to investigate whether the triad of *disease, illness*, and *sickness* remains fruitful in spite of the critique. This will be done by addressing the following questions:

1. What is the triad's explanative power? In particular, how can it be used to analyse controversial cases as well as epistemic and normative challenges to modern medicine?
2. What are the relations among the concepts of the triad? In particular, are any of the concepts primary?
3. Can the concepts of the triad be understood only within the framework of a general theory of *health*, as Nordenfelt claims?
4. Can the triad shed light on why it appears to be so difficult to define basic concepts within modern health care?

---

[2] See for example Bentham 1892; King 1954; Parsons 1951; 1958; Twaddle 1968; Susser 1971; Rothschuh 1972; Frabrega 1972; 1974; 1979; Marinker 1975; Howels 1976; Redlich 1976; Birch 1979; Jenner 1979; Eisenberg & Klienman 1981; Whitbeck 1981; Young 1982; Taylor 1983; Hudson 1983; Twaddle 1993; Nordenfelt 1997/8; Sedgwick 1973; Engelhardt 1995; von Engelhardt 1995.

[3] Nordenfelt applies the term *trichotomy* to describe the relation between disease, illness, and sickness. This seems to have some unfortunate consequences. The word *trichotomy* means divided into three disjoint parts. However, as argued by Twaddle, and as defended in this article, the concepts of disease, illness, and sickness are not exclusive or disjoint. On the contrary, the paradigm case of modern medicine is a member of all three categories. The term *trichotomy* thus misses the point that the concepts of *disease, illness* and *sickness* are not exclusively definable but rather have conjunctive areas. Therefore, the term *trichotomy* is omitted and replaced with the term *triad*.

To address these questions, I will provide a provisional definition of the triad and use it to confront difficult cases discussed in the literature.[4]

Definitions of *disease, illness,* and *sickness*

Since Nordenfelt criticises the definitions of the concepts *disease, illness,* and *sickness* presented by Andrew Twaddle (Twaddle 1973; 1979; 1994a), I will take these definitions as a point of departure.

According to Twaddle, *disease* is defined in the following way: 'Disease is a health problem that consists of a physiological malfunction that results in an actual or potential reduction in physical capacities and/or a reduced life expectancy' (Twaddle 1994a, 8). Ontologically, *disease* is an organic phenomenon, which is comprised of physiological events and independent of subjective experience and social conventions. Epistemically, it is measurable by objective means (Twaddle 1994a, 9).

Illness, by contrast, is defined as follows: 'Illness is a subjectively interpreted undesirable state of health. It consists of subjective feeling states (e.g. pain, weakness), perceptions of the adequacy of their bodily functioning, and/or feelings of competence' (Twaddle 1994a, 10). Ontologically, illness is the subjective feeling of the individual, involving what are often referred to as symptoms. Epistemically, it can only be directly observed by the subject and indirectly accessed through the individual's reports.

Finally, *sickness* is defined as a social identity. 'It is the poor health or the health problem(s) of an individual defined by others with reference to the social activity of that individual' (Twaddle 1994a, 11). Ontologically, Twaddle conceives of *sickness* as 'an event located in society ... defined by participation in the social system' (ibid.). Epistemically, *sickness* is accessed by 'measuring levels of performance with reference to expected social activities when these levels fail to meet social standards ...' (ibid.). *Sickness* is thus a social phenomenon, constituting a new set of rights and duties.

---

[4] Like Nordenfelt's and Twaddle's accounts, the discussion in this chapter is restricted to somatic phenomena. It could be expanded to encompass mental phenomena as well, but that would demand a separate chapter. In addition, the chapter is concerned with the paradigms of the modern Western medical tradition when it refers to the medical profession.

Furthermore, Twaddle outlines the temporal relationship between *disease*, *illness*, and *sickness*. The paradigm case is when a *disease* leads to an *illness*, which then results in *sickness*. Moreover, he gives a relational analysis of the triad in the form of partly overlapping spheres (figure 1)[5].

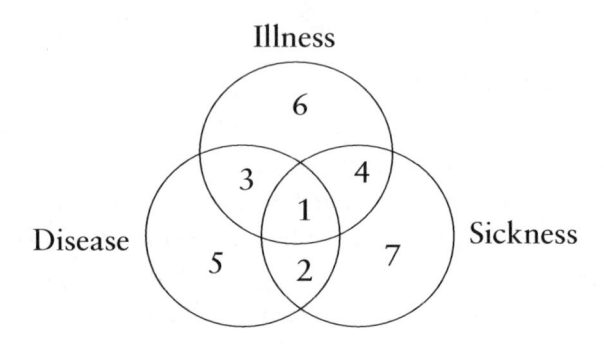

Figure 1: Visual outline of Twaddle's model of the triad. This relationship among the concepts of the triad will be employed in the following analysis.

Deficiencies in Twaddle's triad

The conclusion of Nordenfelt's critical analysis of Twaddle's triad is that it is inadequate to define and describe the condition of 'un-health'. Only within the framework of a general theory of health based on a concept of disability can the triad be fruitful (Nordenfelt 1987, 105–117; 1994, 22, 35). Nordenfelt provides a substantial critique of each member of Twaddle's triad.

Nordenfelt argues that Twaddle's definition of *disease* excludes central phenomena in modern health care. For example, injuries, impairments, and defects reduce human capacities, but they are not obviously encompassed by the definition. According to Nordenfelt, the integration of these categories into the definition of disease has to be based on a concept of health. Furthermore, Nordenfelt focuses on the claim that disease is a 'reduction in physical capacities'. While he appreciates that Twaddle does not refer to a statistical abnormality, he questions whether the 'reduction in physical capacities' is related to the individual. 'Does Twaddle mean that any reduction

---

[5] This figure is essentially identical to Twaddle's (Twaddle 1994a, 15). The layout and numbering is changed here according to the argumentation and structure of this article.

would do, or does he require that the reduction should be of some importance for the individual in question?' (Nordenfelt 1994, 24).

Nordenfelt's dissatisfaction with Twaddle's concept of *illness* contains three aspects. First, together with Wittgenstein and Ryle, he questions whether the subject has any exclusive empirical access to a private mental world. According to Nordenfelt, *illness* is not a hidden private sensation but a perceptible disability. Second, the concept of *illness* as defined is highly diverse. It includes anxiety, pain, itching, lack or loss of competence, and a general feeling of depression (or lack of optimism). According to Nordenfelt, the definition does not provide any means of differentiating between these phenomena, as a health-based concept of *illness* would. Third, the definition of *illness* in terms of the subjective feelings of the individual presupposes that the person is conscious. This is not so in many cases of medical treatment and care. Furthermore, to be able to interpret a state as undesirable implies that the person already possesses the notion of a health problem. Nordenfelt concludes: 'Twaddle has not attempted to give a sharp characterisation of the notion of illness. He has not excluded those undesirable mental states which are obviously not instances of illness' (Nordenfelt 1994, 27).

In the case of *sickness*, Nordenfelt rejects the idea that being sick should be due to a change in activity of the person. There does not need to be any altered activity prior to categorising a person as *sick*. 'The standard case seems to me to be the contrary. There is no particular activity at all, except the seeking of health-care, that could give any clue to the diagnosis concerning the patient' (Nordenfelt 1994, 29). In particular, the paradigm case of declaring a person sick is sick leave, which does not presuppose any such change in social activity on the part of the patient.

According to Nordenfelt, these difficulties show that the triad cannot be meaningful without a general theory of health. His critique of Twaddle, along with Twaddle's answer (Twaddle 1994b), can give the impression that their theories are very far apart. Instead of referring to the detailed discussion between Nordenfelt and Twaddle, I will, for the purposes of this study, only point out some of the similarities between the two.

Twaddle and Nordenfelt revisited

Even though Twaddle and Nordenfelt may have quite different approaches to the conceptual challenges in health care, they seem to have several things in common.

First, Twaddle's triad of *disease, illness,* and *sickness* is related to World Health Organisation's (WHO) definition of health as 'a state of complete physical, psychological and social well-being' (1947). The terms of the triad refer to the spheres of physical, psychological, and social well-being respectively (Twaddle 1994a, 5). Nordenfelt's *welfare* theory of health is also closely related to this definition. He sees health both as the primary concept and as being 'not merely the absence of disease or infirmity' (WHO 1947). Furthermore, the 'ability to realise vital goals' is related to well-being (Nordenfelt 1987, 36). According to Nordenfelt, health is the ability to realise goals which are necessary and together sufficient for a minimal level of happiness (Nordenfelt 1987, 90). At the same time, 'happiness is the most important variant of welfare' (Nordenfelt 1987, 184). Hence, both Twaddle and Nordenfelt relate the basic concepts in health care to welfare.

Second, Twaddle's definitions of *disease, illness,* and *sickness* are based on the notion of *health*. 'Disease is a *health problem*', 'illness is a subjectively interpreted undesirable *state of health*', and sickness is '*poor health* or *health problem(s)* as defined by others' (Twaddle 1994a, 8–11, my emphasis). Thus, the definition of the triad is based on a concept of health (Twaddle 1974; Twaddle 1994b, 51), although it is different from and not as elaborate as Nordenfelt's.[6]

---

[6] Furthermore, it seems worth noting that Nordenfelt actually has only two arguments that support the need for a general theory of health in order to make sense of the triad. First, he argues that the distinctions between disease, defects and injuries can only be made with reference to such a theory. Second, Nordenfelt believes that to be able to make sense of the definition of disease as 'a physiological malfunction that results in an actual or potential reduction in physical capacities and/or reduced life expectancy', one needs a general theory of health (Nordenfelt 1994, 24). However, he does not give any clear arguments for this latter claim. Twaddle can still claim that cases of defects and injuries are part of diseases and that his definition of disease holds without referring to health. The argument of this chapter, however, is that this is possible without any elaborated theory of health.

Third, Twaddle's primary concept is *sickness*. *Disease* and *illness* are mainly of interest in so far as they result in *sickness*. Similarly, Nordenfelt's primary concept of 'un-health' is *disability*. *Disease*, *defects*, and *injuries* are conditions that may lead to *disability*, and they are of interest only in so far as they do. This certainly allows for comparison between the two, and Twaddle himself notes: 'Nordenfelt seems to be bringing his concept of disability very close to my concept of sickness' (Twaddle 1994b, 50). Nordenfelt's 'non-capacity of performing a set of activities given standard circumstances' (Nordenfelt 1994, 29) is similar to Twaddle's definition of *sickness* as an inability to perform expected social activities (Twaddle 1994a, 11). This similarity is confirmed by Twaddle's concept of health which takes into account the 'individual's capacities for task or role performance' (Twaddle 1974, 31). Thus, there is a close relationship between Nordenfelt's concept of ability and Twaddle's concept of capacity and between Nordenfelt's concept of disability and Twaddle's concept of sickness. Furthermore, as will be discussed later in this chapter, the concepts of *sickness* and *disability* both have epistemic and normative dimensions.

Thus, despite the differences, there are basic similarities in their perspectives. Does this imply that it is possible to reconcile Nordenfelt's and Twaddle's concepts of the triad? Is it possible, on the basis of their discussion, to give strict and consistent definitions of the concepts of *disease*, *illness*, and *sickness*? Although Nordenfelt's and Twaddle's conceptions might not be so different after all, and it may be tempting to tinker with the definitions so as to render them more consistent and concordant, this chapter will not pursue that task. There has been a comprehensive debate on the basic concepts of health care from a variety of perspectives.[7] The concepts of *disease*, *illness*, and *sickness* are widely recognised in the literature, but they are subject to substantial controversy. Since the objective of this chapter is to investigate the fruitfulness of the triad, I will not enter into this extensive and complex debate. Instead, only a coarse and tentative definition of the triad, disease, illness, and sickness will be given in order to investigate its explanatory power.

---

[7] For example from the realist or nominalist perspective (King 1954; Cohen 1961; Rather 1958; Scadding 1967; Rothschuh 1972; Kennedy 1981; Gillon 1986; Sundström 1987); analytic or holistic (Nordenfelt 1987); naturalist or normativist (Reznek 1987; Räikkä 1997; Kovács 1998); objectivist or subjectivist (Lennox 1995; Sade 1995; Kovács 1998), ontological or physiological (Rather 1958; Temkin 1963; Hudson 1983) theoretical or practical (Boorse 1977; Jensen 1984; Brown 1985; Hesslow 1993) or value-laden or value free (Margolis 1976; Boorse 1975; Turner 1987; Fulford 1993).

Disease, illness, and *sickness* as different perspectives

The concepts of *disease, illness*, and *sickness* emphasise different perspectives on important aspects of human life. The concepts of *disease, illness*, and *sickness* reflect professional, personal, and social perspectives respectively and, further, they concern biological, phenomenological, and behavioural phenomena. This has become widely accepted in the literature and in practice. Furthermore, *disease, illness*, and *sickness* are negative notions reflecting occurrences in human life of negative value.

Moreover, each concept calls for action. *Disease* calls for actions by the medical profession with the goals of identifying and treating the occurrence and caring for the person. *Illness* changes the actions of the individual, making one communicate one's personal perspective on the negative occurrence to others by, for example, calling for help. *Sickness* calls for a determination of the social status of the sick person, in particular, deciding who is entitled to treatment and economic rights and who is to be exempted from social duties, such as work.

The main point here is not to enter into the vast, vivid, and multifaceted debate on the definition of these concepts, but to investigate their fruitfulness. Therefore, it suffices here to point out that they represent different perspectives on human aliment, i.e., professional, personal, and social perspectives. Indeed, strict definitions of the concepts might even leave out important explanatory aspects and restrict their fruitfulness.

The triad in practice: comprising controversial cases

How then can coarse conceptions of *disease, illness*, and *sickness* be of any value? In the discussion on the basic concepts of health care, practical cases have been employed to evaluate the definitions of the concepts. 'Descriptive' or 'naturalist' theories have been accused of making pregnancy, excellence, and homosexuality into diseases. On the other hand, 'normativist' or 'nominalist' theories are charged with making ageing and general dissatisfaction diseases.[8] In the following, I will try to analyse the triad with respect to such controversial cases to investigate the fruitfulness of the perspectivistic distinction between *disease*, *illness*, and *sickness*.

The paradigm case in health care is when a person feels *ill*, the medical profession is able to detect *disease*, and society attributes to him the status of being *sick*. *Illness* explains the person's situation to himself, *disease* permits medical attention, and *sickness* frees him from ordinary duties of work and gives him the right to economic assistance (area 1 in Figure 1). Examples of such conditions are numerous. There appears to be agreement about conditions such as myocardial infarction, tuberculosis, and renal failure. Negative bodily occurrences as conceived of by the individual correspond with negative bodily occurrences recognised by the medical profession and by relevant social institutions.

Thus, cases of *disease*, *illness*, and *sickness* are paradigms of health care. There are, however, several other conditions deviating from this ideal, that is, conditions in which only two members of the triad are relevant.

There are instances of conditions which satisfy the criteria for both *disease* and *sickness*, but not for *illness* (2). For example, there are conditions in which certain signs or markers are recognised by the medical profession before the patient experiences any illness, and, as a result of which, society entitles the person to treatment and economic support. High blood pressure (without symptoms), hepatitis G, human papilloma virus (HPV), ductal carcinoma in situ (DCIS), and other conditions subject to screening and predictive testing belong to this group. The professionals are confident that they are dealing with *disease*, social institutions designate the person in question as *sick*, but that person is not *ill*. The same situation can be recognised when patients are unconscious or have impairments recognised by the medical profession and by society, but not by the person in question.

There are also cases which are instances of both *disease* and *illness*, but not of *sickness* (3). Examples are the common cold, tooth decay, ageing, and

---

[8] Nordenfelt tries to avoid this objection by excluding from illness emotions which are direct reactions to external events (Nordenfelt 1987, 114–7). This seems difficult in practice. How are we to know what is caused by external events? Furthermore, what is the difference between the grief experienced when losing (the sensation in) a leg and that of losing a close relatives?

seasickness.[9] The medical profession is able to recognise these conditions as *disease* by various diagnostic measures and the person in question certainly experiences them as such, but they normally do not qualify as *sickness*.

Furthermore, there are conditions which are both *illness* and *sickness* but not *disease* (4). Fibromyalgia, low back pain, whiplash, and chronic fatigue syndrome are examples of conditions in which the person certainly feels ill and society entitles the person to have the status of being *sick*, but the medical profession cannot always identify or detect *disease*. Correspondingly, pregnancy is commonly not conceived of as *disease* by the medical profession, although it might be experienced by many women as *illness* and accepted by society as a reason for *sickness*.[10]

Another group of cases covers conditions in which only one of the concepts of the triad is relevant. Asymptomatic instances of hyperglycaemia, hypertension (low or moderate), and lactose intolerance (in areas where people do not normally drink milk) are examples of *disease* which are neither *illness* nor *sickness* (5). The medical profession conceives of these and diagnoses them as *disease*, but the person does not experience them as such and they do not normally qualify as *sickness*.

Correspondingly, instances of *illness* which are neither *disease* nor *sickness* (6) represent cases that are experienced by the person as negative, but are not recognised as *disease* by the medical profession or as *sickness* by society. A general feeling of dissatisfaction, unpleasantness, incompetence, anxiety, and melancholia might be examples.

The last group concerning only one of the triad's concepts are cases of *sickness*, which are neither *disease* nor *illness* (7). Delinquency, dissidence, homosexuality, skin colour, and masturbation may count as examples of cases in which social institutions have designated people as *sick*, but the person has not felt ill and the medical profession has not diagnosed any negative bodily correlates.[11]

---

[9] It might rightly be argued that seasickness is a *sickness* if one is a member of a boat crew. However, for many boat crews, seasickness does not qualify one for sick leave. Rather, it is stigmatising, calling into question one's identity as a member of the boat crew.

[10] It is interesting to note that because pregnancy is conceived of as both *illness* and *sickness*, it is made the subject of the health care system, even though it is not recognised by the medical profession as a *disease*.

[11] The examples of *sickness*, but not *illness* or *disease* are mainly historical examples, as we like to believe that today's society is free of such repressive actions. In Norway, however,

Thus, the triad appears to be able to account for controversial cases discussed in the literature. The claim here is neither that these are the only possible examples nor that the cases cannot be interpreted otherwise but that the concepts of *disease*, *illness*, and *sickness* represent a framework for understanding the controversial cases.

Additionally, the triad provides the tools for an analysis of some of the controversies in the debates on human ailment. In the next section, some of the epistemic and normative challenges in medicine will be investigated on the basis of the triad.

Epistemic and normative consequences

Several interesting observations, with both epistemic and normative implications, follow from the above analysis. Cases incorporating *disease*, *illness*, and *sickness* (1) are neither epistemically nor normatively problematic. The person experiences a negative bodily occurrence making him request help, the medical profession recognises certain signs and knows what can be done, and society and its institutions entitle him to treatment, economic support, and freedom from certain obligations like work.

The three kinds of cases, in which only one member of the triad is applicable (5, 6, and 7), are quite challenging. First, when the medical profession classifies a condition as a *disease*, but the patient does not feel any *illness* and society does not find any reason to change his or her social status (5), both epistemic and normative difficulties result. How can we know that people with asymptomatic diseases will actually develop symptoms and become ill? Should people with low or moderate hypertension be subject to extensive treatment? Is sickle cell trait a matter of medical concern in areas with malaria? Can it be right to treat polydactylism and obesity if it does not bother the person? Here we encounter ethical issues related to patient autonomy, paternalism, and liberty.[12]

---

the government tries to make the medical profession perform tests (genetic and x-ray) on asylum seekers, to investigate whether they have the sickness of 'lying about their identity'.
[12] If the medical profession is the only one identifying *disease*, their sensitivity to the interests of the person and society, will determine whether they act paternalistic or violate patient autonomy. Additionally, one can question how well a person without *illness* understands information about diseases that he or she cannot experience. Is there a real informed consent?

Second, situations in which a person is suffering (there is *illness*) but no *disease* has been found and there is no change in one's social status (6) also represent epistemic and normative challenges. Epistemically, it is difficult for the medical profession to discover the cause of the suffering. Normatively, it is hard to see what society ought to do in such situations. A general feeling of dissatisfaction does not normally qualify the person for medical care or economic support. On the other hand, medical intervention has been initiated in such cases and has been criticised for being medicalising. Trying to handle all cases of illness is also a matter of resources and hence a question of prioritisation.

Third, cases of *sickness* which are neither *disease* nor *illness* (7) are challenging and might even be dangerous. Skin colour, drapetomania (a 'disease' that made slaves run away), masturbation, homosexuality, and political dissidence are crude examples. There appears to be no professionally accepted diagnostic criteria in these cases. Further, the norms that have been appealed to in order to entitle a person to be *sick* in these cases have later been found to be dubious.

While cases in which only one member of the triad is applicable certainly call for special attention, cases in which two are pertinent (2, 3, and 4) *may be* epistemically and normatively challenging as well. First, cases of both *disease* and *illness* but not of *sickness* (3) are subject to pressure from professionals and interest groups for support. There may be several reasons why the status of *sickness* is not granted, even though the person has both *disease* and *illness*. There can be a lack of resources, the situation may be common or equally distributed in a population, or there might be no cure available. Myopia and tooth decay are examples of cases that are not conceived of as *sickness* in many countries, but are acknowledged to be *disease* by the medical profession and experienced negatively by persons with these conditions. The epistemic challenge is to find effective and efficient cures, whereas the normative challenges are connected to questions of rationing and to cases in which people are not able to pay for health care services themselves.

Second, cases of both *illness* and *sickness* but not of *disease* (4) put pressure on the medical research community to find mechanisms and causes of these occurrences, which are both personally experienced and economically supported. Fibromyalgia, whiplash, and low back pain are examples. The aetiology of and treatment for these conditions are not commonly agreed upon. They have, however, been accepted in various countries as *sickness*, and people certainly claim to experience them as *illness*. There is pressure on the medical establishment to see these conditions as *disease* as well. There is both an epistemic challenge to establish aetiology and a normative challenge to find a treatment, since such conditions ought to be treated.

Third, cases of both *disease* and *sickness* which are not *illness* (2) generate some profound challenges. Epistemically, we are challenged by the question of whether general knowledge applies to this particular person, that is, how certain we can be that the person actually will become *ill* when test results indicate *disease*. Many cases of *disease* will not develop to *illness* if left untreated (Feinstein 1967; Fischer & Welch 1999). Normatively, we are faced with a series of questions: How are we to handle the results from predictive testing? Are there limits to the treatment of asymptomatic diseases? How are we to break the bad news? The discussion on genetic testing, hypercholesterolaemia, and hypertension illustrates some of these normative challenges (Le Fanu 1999). How far can we go in treatment of cases in which the patient is not *ill*? How is patient autonomy preserved? Who is to determine the trade-off between the risks and the benefit of such treatment? These conditions touch on some of the most intensively discussed controversies in modern medical ethics and raise questions about patient autonomy, paternalism, and medicalisation.

Hence, cases which fall under only one or two of the concepts represent epistemic and normative challenges as well. The above discussion indicates that the concepts of *disease*, *illness*, and *sickness* represent a fruitful framework for analysing some of the pressing epistemic and normative problems of modern medicine.

Differences between the areas (1–7)

From the discussion above, it can be argued that cases which belong to only one of the spheres of the triad may be more challenging than cases which belong to two. We appear to be more challenged by medical treatment of incompetence, dissatisfaction, homosexuality, dissidence, and low or moderate hyperglycaemia than we are by the treatment of asymptomatic breast cancer, common colds, and seasickness.

Cases are stronger and less controversial if they are recognised by two of the agents as being both *disease* and *sickness* (2), both *disease* and *illness* (3), or both *illness* and *sickness* (4) than if they are only recognised by one of the agents as *disease* (5), *illness* (6), or *sickness* (7). People, professionals, or social institutions appear to have a weaker case, if the condition belongs to only one sphere. The pressure on medicine to accept an occurrence as *disease* is strong when it is recognised both as *illness* and *sickness*. In the same way, there is pressure on society to provide necessary resources and to admit that an occurrence is *sickness* when it is recognised both as *disease* and *illness*.

In cases of only *illness*, the ill person has to convince both the medical profession and social institutions about his or her situation. Similarly, social institutions have to convince both the medical profession and the person in cases of *sickness* alone, and both society and the person have to be persuaded in cases of only *disease*. Thus, cases in which only member of the triad is applicable appear to be difficult.

Thus, there are normative and epistemic differences among the areas (1–7) whereby membership of only one sphere is more challenging than membership of two. In order to find directions for what *to do*, I will investigate the normative differences between the areas in further detail in the following section.

The primacy of *illness*

One interesting observation resulting from the analysis of the triad of *disease*, *illness*, and *sickness* is the difference in challenges between these conjunctive areas. Area (2) seems to cause more challenges than areas (3) and (4). Conditions like fibromyalgia, whiplash, and low back pain (4) seem mainly to challenge the medical profession (in lack of knowledge and treatment). Cases of the common cold, tooth decay, warts, and lung and throat irritations due to cigarette smoking (3) primarily challenge the resources of the society in question. A predominant proportion of medical ethics cases seems to concern cases of *disease* and *sickness* but not *illness* (2). To treat people when they do not know that they need help appears to represent a major challenge to modern health care. Issues of patient autonomy, paternalism, and medicalisation belong to this area.

Accordingly, we appear to be more willing to accept cases of only *illness* (6) than those of only *disease* (5) or of only *sickness* (7). For example, it seems easier for us to accept giving people treatment and care in cases where there are no medical indications in terms of *disease* (6) than to treat people against their knowledge or will (5, 7). The first case is a matter of limited medical knowledge and recourses. However, treatment in cases of only *disease* (5) or of only *sickness* (6) raises more profound issues, such as patient autonomy, paternalism, and medicalisation, and these cases appear to be more challenging.

Hence, the most challenging cases appear to be those of *disease* and *sickness* (2), those of only *disease* (5), and those of only *sickness* (6). What does this tell us? Common to these cases is that they lack *illness*. This must mean that the most profound challenges that are related to the triad of *disease*, *illness*, and *sickness* are to be found in cases without *illness*. That is, there appears to be an epistemic and normative primacy of the concept of illness. This accords well with a substantial critique of modern medicine directed at its ignorance of the subjective experience of the individual patient, i.e. of *illness*.[13] It also agrees with the epistemic-normative foundation of medicine evident from antiquity until today: the primacy of the individual person who is ill.[14]

What consequences does the primacy of *illness* have for health care? Does it result in an overall subjective approach? Does it make any kind of ailment a case to be treated by the health care system or to deserve exemption from social duties?[15] This certainly does not seem to be the case. Within the framework of the triad, the categories of *disease* and *sickness* limit the situations of *illness* to be handled by the health care system. The triad provides a framework for acknowledging people's *illness*. At the same time, the triad reveals that health care professionals cannot and should not identify *disease* in all instances of *illness*. Similarly, the analysis of the triad articulates society's abridged ability to ascribe *sickness* to a person in all cases of *illness*.

---

[13] See e.g. Illich 1975; Knowles 1977; Reiser 1978; Pellegrino & Thomasma 1981; 1993; Jonas 1985; Beauchamp & Childress 1989; Gadamer 1993; Delkeskamp-Hayes & Cutter 1993; Tyreman 2006.

[14] Furthermore, in the practical taxonomy of medicine, there is an extensive class of symptomatic diseases. Although the aetiology is unknown and there are no clinical or paraclinical signs, they are classified and handled by the medical profession as diseases. There is a corresponding conception of *disease* without *illness* and sickness, e.g., lanthanic disease or psuedudisease (Feinstein 1976; Fischer & Welch 1999). However, they are not subject to similar attention as symptoms-based diseases.

[15] An interesting case illustrates this. The son of a well known bishop had lost several millions NOK in gambling. This was money he had 'borrowed' from his parents in order to finance his business, alleged to be in a critical phase. The parents had borrowed the money from friends. As the son lost the money, the parents went bankrupt, and he was sentenced to four years in prison. However, in the appeal case they argued that he had a disease (velokardiofacial syndrome) that did cause his actions, and that should reduce his sentence significantly.

Illness, then, without *disease* and/or *sickness*, is challenging and must be 'handled with care'. The very existence of *illness* can be taken seriously and examined cautiously both by the medical profession and by the appropriate social institutions. It does not, however, automatically qualify one for help from the health care system. This will be determined by whether negative bodily occurrence can be identified by the medical profession (*disease*) and by relevant social institutions (*sickness*).

It is worth noting that within a system based on the concept of *health*, as suggested by Nordenfelt, one has to rely on special restrictions like, for example, statistical normality or external events (Nordenfelt 1987, 114–7). Otherwise, all cases of *illness* become eligible for treatment by the health care system, including, for example, incompetence and general dissatisfaction. Nordenfelt tries to restrict the concept of *illness* from within the concept itself, and he does this by making qualifications that are external to the person experiencing illness. This approach appears to be problematic. The triad, on the other hand, acknowledges illness as the negative bodily occurrences experienced by the person in question and classifies the cases that are to be subject to medical treatment as *disease* and those that are to gain economic support as *sickness*. This suggests that the triad is more robust with regard to the threat of 'subjectivism' (Lennox 1995; Sade 1995; Kovács 1998; Edwards 1998) than a health based system.

The primacy of *illness* should not come as a surprise. If the moral basis of health care is to help people, then it follows that the help should be given in ways that can be experienced by the people receiving the health care. If the health care intervention cannot be experienced by the person, in terms of survival and reduced morbidity, symptoms, or pain, then it becomes challenging to justify the intervention.

The triad and the concept of health – or: why we do not need a concept of health in order to treat disease

The tentative account of the triad given above is dependent only on the professional, personal, and social perspectives of human ailment and not on a positive conception or theory of health. The triad of *disease*, *illness*, and *sickness* has been shown to serve a practical purpose in understanding 'controversial cases' and to present a framework for analysing epistemic and normative challenges to medicine. Furthermore, the analysis has revealed normative differences between the members of the triad and, in particular, the primacy of the concept of *illness*. Hence, the triad has been shown to be fruitful without a concept of health.

This conclusion coincides with Tranøy's argument that we are more ready to define negative notions such as *illness* and *disease* than *health* (Tranøy 1967, 355). Tranøy relates this point to a general asymmetry in ethics. There is a higher "moral weight" attached to negative notions than to positive ones. There is an asymmetry between concepts such as *good* and *bad*, *health* and *disease*, or *life* and *death* (Tranøy 1967, 351). Hans Georg Gadamer's general emphasis on negative critique (Gadamer 1960) seems to support this idea. In particular, it is in accordance with his characterization of the hiddenness or enigma of health (*Die Verborgenheit der Gesundheit*) (Gadamer 1993). Gadamer argues that *health*, as the aim of medicine, is not a definable concept. Ailment (Krankheit), however, is. Furthermore, he acknowledges the professional, personal, and social aspects of human ailment, as well as their normative aspects (Gadamer 1987, 258).[16]

This is not the proper place to enter into a detailed discussion on asymmetries in ethics. Suffice it here to note that the triad has been employed without a general theory of health and that it has been fruitful to analyse important epistemic and normative challenges to modern medicine. Hence, we do not need a concept of health in order to handle people's negative bodily occurrences. To further illustrate the triad's fruitfulness, let me turn to the last question raised at the outset of this chapter: how can the triad explain the difficulties of defining the basic concepts of health care?

Difficulties of definition

Conditions such as pregnancy, excellence, ageing, fibromyalgia, homosexuality, a general feeling of dissatisfaction, and incompetence have challenged explicit definitions of basic concepts of health care. Biostatistical definitions have been profoundly challenged by conditions such as pregnancy, excellence,

---

[16] '[t]he goal of health is not a condition that is clearly deniable from within the medical art. For illness is a social state of affairs, much more than a fact that is determinable from within the natural sciences' (Gadamer 1996, 20).

and homosexuality because they represent deviance from statistical 'normality'. Welfare-based definitions (well-being, happiness, goal-realisation, action failure) are challenged by the conditions of dissatisfaction and incompetence, because these tend to relativise the concepts.

In order to handle these difficulties, many have tried to refine the definitions of the basic concepts of health care. However, as it has been argued here, there appear to be distinct perspectives on occurrences which are conceived of as human ailment. To embrace all these perspectives in one single concept appears to be difficult.

Furthermore, some of the definitions of basic concepts in modern health care appear to be monistic (i.e., reduced to a single phenomenon, theory, or perspective). Although there is a variety of basic concepts in health care, such as *health*, *disease*, *illness*, and *sickness*, one single concept is the basic concept from which the other concepts are derived. For example, Nordenfelt derives concepts like *disease* and *illness* from his concept of *health*. Again, a monistic approach appears to face the same challenges of taking into account the different perspectives and trying to account for all of them with one concept.

In addition, the debates on the concepts of human ailment (e.g. on *disease*) run into deep and apparently irresolvable philosophical issues that may be difficult to reconcile in an encompassing definition (Hofmann 2001). Strategies to define diseases may be based on unsound philosophical conceptions, such as the analytic-synthetic distinction (Nordby 2006). Nevertheless, definitions of basic concepts of human ailment for use in restricted fields may in principle be possible and even fruitful (Hofmann 2010).

The difficulties of defining the basic concepts are not only due to the described complexity of perspectives but also to the relations among them. *Disease*, *illness*, and *sickness* are not static concepts, they influence each other, and the borders between them are blurred. This influence can be described in three different ways.

Interrelating concepts

First, the concepts of *disease*, *illness*, and *sickness* are not independent of each other. The attribution of a social status (*sickness*) is influenced by distinctions made, processes described, and entities applied in the medical profession. *Infertility*, traditionally not considered a *sickness*, qualifies for economic support in many countries because it has become treatable as a *disease*. On the other hand, it is argued that infertility is a *disease* because that renders it *sickness*, i.e., covered by health insurance.

Similarly, the experience of *illness* is affected by medical knowledge. The personal experience of ailment is influenced by the medical terminology, e.g. a soccer player might state that he has some pain in his *meniscus*, or a patient can feel his 'large intestines a bit bound' (Nessa & Malterud 1998). New imaging techniques may also influence both *illness* and *disease* (Kevles 1997; McCabe & Castel 2008). Conversely, the experience of *illness* influences the activities of the medical profession. Research into lower back pain and whiplash was initiated by peoples' suffering and need for help. The status of pregnancy and childbirth as *illnesses* and *sicknesses* has made the medical establishment hospitalise pregnant women as if they were having *disease*.[17]

Correspondingly, the professionals preoccupied with *disease* are influenced by the social status of *sickness*. Disease entities vary greatly in social status and prestige (Album and Westin 2008). The search for a causal explanation for fibromyalgia is supported by its status as *illness* and *sickness*. On the other hand, cases of the common cold are not usually classified as *sickness*; therefore, the viruses which are the etiologic agents are normally not traced, even though this is technologically possible (Copeland 1977, 530). Furthermore, the social sphere governs medical education and research to a large extent. The social and psychological influences on the concept of disease are clearly reflected in the influential biopsychosocial model of disease (Engel 1977).

Second, the class membership of the areas may vary over time. As Twaddle already pointed out, a person may be a member of none, one or more of the concepts at the same time (Twaddle 1994a, 13–16). Even more, the membership may be complex and change with time, e.g. both the medical professionals and ill people are members of society, and thus all influence the sphere of *sickness*. In particular, in some countries, the physician is the representative of society and manages both *disease* and *sickness* at the same time.[18] Furthermore, all members of society, whether medical professionals or not, may become *ill*.

---

[17] Furthermore, if the differentiations between disease entities are of no influence on the *illness* of patients, they are in practice abandoned, e.g. the histopathological distinction between meningothelial type I and type II meningiomas is seldom made. Both tumours share the same prognosis and treatment (Copeland 1977, 535–6).

[18] This is particularly so in the Scandinavian health care system, in which physicians administer sick leave, making them directly involved in the sphere of *sickness*, in addition to that of *disease*.

That is, infection with human papilloma virus (HPV) may at one point be only *disease*, but later be *disease* and *sickness*, dependant on the knowledge of the relationship between HPV and cervix cancer as well as breast cancer.

Third, a practical-historical observation may be added. The concept of disease changes with time, depends on praxis, and influences medical taxonomy. Diseases are defined according to abnormalities of morphology, physiological aberrations, biochemical defects, genetic abnormalities, ultrastuctural abnormalities, and etiologic agents (Copeland 1977, 530). Hence, it has been difficult to provide a consistent medical taxonomy. There is no unified nosology (ibid.), and the taxonomy seems to be more influenced by prognostic and therapeutic capacity than by formal definitions (Scadding 1967).[19]

In the next chapter (chapter 2) I will elaborate even further on the dynamics of the basic concepts of human ailment, in particular on the concept of *sickness*.

Thus, the distinctions between *disease*, *illness*, and *sickness* are not clearcut. Twaddle's ideal relation of *disease* leading to *illness* subsequently resulting in *sickness* appears too simplistic, and Nordenfelt's conception of them as disjoint (as a trichotomy) seems to be difficult to defend. As argued, the concepts are not disjoint, but the borders between them are blurred, and the concepts influence each other. *Disease, illness*, and *sickness* are thus interdependent concepts.

Though concepts of the triad are concerned with the same matter, namely, human ailment in terms of negative occurrences (bodily or mentally), the extensions of *disease, illness*, and *sickness* relate to different perspectives. This might be why it appears to be difficult to give one assembling definition of all negative bodily occurrences, or why it is so difficult to define them in terms of each other (Hofmann 2005).[20] Thus, the interrelated but different perspectives represent an inherent difficulty in providing strictly consistent definitions, and this may explain why the definitions of basic concepts such as *disease, illness*, and *sickness* have become controversial in the philosophy of medicine.

---

[19] Additionally, at a given point in history, there is not always agreement regarding what is *disease* and what is *sickness* within the medical profession and the social institutions respectively.

[20] Tranøy has pointed out that some of the basic concepts of health care, such as *health* and *disease*, belong to different categories and thus are not definable by each other. Although they are interdependent, they are not interdefinable (Tranøy 1995a; 1995b).

Concluding remarks

The point of departure for this chapter was a review of the debate between Twaddle and Nordenfelt on the triad *disease*, *illness*, and *sickness*. It acknowledged Nordenfelt's critique of Twaddle's definitions, but instead of tinkering with these definitions in order to render them less objectionable, a coarse and tentative account that acknowledged the different perspectives on human ailment (professional, personal, and social) was taken as the point of departure.

The objective has been to investigate whether the triad, *disease*, *illness*, and *sickness* still can be fruitful, and in particular, to investigate its explanatory power. Some conclusions can been drawn from this analysis:

First, the triad of *disease*, *illness*, and *sickness* is able to address controversies over basic concepts in health care. It is thus a suitable conceptual framework for analysing and facing controversial cases. In particular, the triad represents a framework for addressing the normative as well as the epistemic challenges in medicine. It enables us to identify and analyse normative matters such as autonomy, paternalism, rationing, and medicalisation in terms of conflicting perspectives.

Second, the analysis also reveals epistemic and normative differences between the concepts, in particular, the primacy of *illness*. This is in accordance with a common account in the philosophy of medicine. It does not, however, imply that all cases of *illness* are to be treated by the health care system. The other spheres of the triad, *disease* and *sickness*, protect society from medicalisation of the life world. Not all *illness* is the concern of medicine, nor is happiness its goal.

Third, the triad of *disease*, *illness*, and *sickness* can be fruitful without a general concept of health. We do not need a concept of health to respond to human ailment. In particular, we do not need a concept of health to treat disease. This agrees with the philosophical account that ailment is more easy to conceive of than health, due to the general primacy of negative normative notions to positive ones.

Fourth, it has been argued that the triad explains why it is so difficult to render strict and consistent definitions of concepts such as *disease*, *illness*, and *sickness*. These concepts are not mutually exclusive but, rather, interdependent.

They represent different perspectives on human ailment and are thus difficult to unite in a strict and consistent definition.

Another commonplace but significant conclusion can be added: since it has been argued that the triad of *disease, illness,* and *sickness* is fruitful without a conceptual framework of health, the term 'health care' appears to be a paradox. A consequence of this analysis is that it seems to be both difficult and unnecessary to define the concepts of *disease, illness,* and *sickness* in terms of *health*. Thus, a system or institution intended to handle cases of human ailment does not properly fall under the term '*health* care', thus 'health care' is a contradictory term since the attention is directed at eliminating human ailment and not at the promotion of health.[21] To avoid the paradox of 'health care' and to include the structures of the triad, it might be more proper to differentiate between a *disease treatment system,* an *illness care system,* and a *sickness rights system.* Instead of trying to save the term 'health care' by elaborating a system of 'health enhancement' (Nordenfelt 1998), the ailment-based triad restricts the duties and rights in a medical system. There is a fundamental difference between a 'health care system' based on negative notions of human ailment such as *disease, illness,* and *sickness* and a system based on the concept of *health*.

A clearer differentiation of what is called 'health care' appears to be fruitful. The concepts of the triad exhibit profound perspectives on human ailment. The medical profession provides a perspective that is different from that of the patient and from that of social institutions. It is because *disease* is distinct from both *illness* and *sickness* that the medical profession is able to help. This means, however, that *illness* or *sickness* cannot be reduced to *disease*. That is, there are limits to what the medical profession can be expected to do and what it should do. Similarly, the other concepts of the triad represent distinct subject matters with characteristic limitations. Hence, the concepts of the triad display profound limitations that are easily neglected in the 'health care' system.

---

[21] Even Nordenfelt's health-based concept seems to suffer from this paradox. In his analysis of general health enhancement, he returns to defining medical care in terms of disease and injuries. Medical care aims at 'eradicating diseases and injuries by cure or at reducing the negative consequences of diseases and injuries for the person who has been stricken' (Nordenfelt 1998, 75). If health really had primacy in relation to *disease, illness* and *sickness* (including defects and injuries), then a system of health enhancement should not need to be based on 'medical care' dealing with ailment. Furthermore, a definition of medical *care* should not need to be based on the *treatment of disease*.

Acknowledgement

This chapter is a revised version of the article, 'On the triad disease, illness and sickness' which was published in volume 27, number 6 of the *Journal of Medicine and Philosophy* in 2002 (pages 651–74), published by Oxford University Press.

References

Album D. & S. Westin 2008. 'Do diseases have a prestige hierarchy? A survey among physicians and medical students'. *Social Science and Medicine* 66(1), 182–188

Beachamp T.L. & J.F. Childress 1989. *Principles of Biomedicla Ethics*. New York, Oxford University Press

Boorse, C. 1975. 'On the Distincion Between Disease and Illness'. *Philosophy and Public Affairs* 5, 49–68

Boorse, C. 1977. 'Health as a Theoretical Concept'. *Philosophy of science* 44, 542–573

Brown, W.M. 1985. 'On Defining 'Disease'. *Journal of Medicine and Philosophy* 10, 311–28

Cohen, H. 1961. 'The evolution of the concept of disease'. Lush, B. ed.: *Concepts of Medicine: a collection of essays on aspects of medicine.* Oxford, Pergamon Press

Copeland, D.D. 1977. 'Concepts of Disease and Diagnosis'. *Persp Biol Med* 20, 528–38

Crombie, A.C. ed. 1963. *Scientific Change: Historical Studies in the Intellectual, Social and Technical Conditions for Scientific Discovery and Technical Invention from Antiquity to the Present.* New York, Basic Books, 629–47

Delkeskamp-Hayes, C. & M.A.G Cutter 1993. *Science, technology, and the art of medicine: European-American dialogues*. Dordrecht, Kluwer Academic

Eisenberg, L. & A. Kleinman 1981. *The Relevance of Social Science for Medicine*. Dortrecht, Reidel

Engel, G.L. 1977. 'The need for a new medical model: A challenge for biomedicine'. *Science* 196, 129–36

Engelhardt, H.T. 1975. 'The concepts of health and disease'. Engehlardt, H T & S F Spicker eds.: *Evaluation and explanation in the biomedical sciences*. Dordrecht, Reidel, 125–41

Engehlardt, H.T. & S.F. Spicker eds. 1975. *Evaluation and explanation in the biomedical sciences*. Dordrecht, Reidel

Feinstein, A.R. 1967. *Clinical Judgement*. Baltimore, The Williams and Wilkins Company

Fischer, E.S. & H.G. Welch 1999. Avoiding the Unintended Consequences of Growth in Medical Care'. *JAMA* 281, 446–53

Fulford, K.W.M 1993. 'Praxis makes perfect: Illness as a bridge between biological concepts of disease and social conceptions of health'. *Theoretical Medicine* 14, 305–20

Gadamer, H.G. 1960. *Wahrheit und Methode: Grundzüge einer philosophischen Hermeneutik*. Tübringen, Mohr

Gadamer, H.G. 1987. *Gesammelte Werke*. Tübringen, Mohr, Vol.4

Gadamer, H.G. 1993. *Über die Verborgenheit der Gesundheit*. Frankfurt am Main, Suhrkamp

Gadamer, H.G. 1996. *The Enigma of Health: The Art of Healing in a Scientific Age*. Translated by Jason Gaiger and Nicholas Walker. Stanford, California, Stanford University Press

Gillon, R. 1986. 'On sickness and on helath'. *Brit Med J* 292, 318–20

Hesslow, G. 1993. 'Do we need a concept of disease?'. *Theoretical Medicine* 14, 1–14

Hofmann B. 2001. 'Complexity of the concept of disease as shown through rival theoretical frameworks'. *Theoretical Medicine and Bioethics* 22(3), 211–37

Hofmann B. 2005. 'Simplified models of the relationship between health and disease'. *Theoretical Medicine and Bioethics* 26(5), 355–77

Hofmann B. 2010. 'The concept of disease – vague, complex, polyvalent, or just indefinable?' *Med Health Care and Philos* 13, 3–10

Hudson, R.P. 1983. *Disease and its Control*. London, Greenwood Press

Illich, I. 1975. *Medical Nemesis : The Expropriation of Health*. Calder and Boyars, London

Jaco, E.G. ed. 1958. *Patients, physicians and illness : sourcebook in behavioral science and medicine*. New York, Free Press

Jensen, U.J. 1984. 'A critique of essentialism in medicine'. Nordenfelt, L. & B.I.B. Lindahl eds.: *Health, disease and causal explanations in medicine*. Boston, Reidel, 63–3

Jonas, H. 1985. *Technik, Medizin und Ethik*. Frankfurt am Main, Insel Verlag
Kennedy, I. 1983. *The Unmasking of Medicine*. London, Granada
Kevles B. 1997. *Naked to the bone: medical imaging in the twentieth century*. New Brunswick NJ, Rutgers University Press
King, L. 1954. 'What is a Disease?'. *Philosophy of Science* 21, 193–203
Knowles, J.H. ed. 1977. *Doing better and feeling worse*. New York, Norton & Co.
Kovács, J. 1998. 'The concept of health and disease'. *Medicine, Health Care and Philosophy* 1, 31–9
Le Fanu, J. 1999. *The rise and fall of modern medicine*. London, Little Brown
Lennox, J. 1995. 'Health as an objective value'. *Journal of Medicine and Philosophy* 20, 499–511
Liss, P.E. & B. Petersson eds. 1995. *Helsosamma tankar*. Nora, Nya Doxa
Lush, B. ed. 1961. *Concepts of Medicine: a collection of essays on aspects of medicine*. Oxford, Pergamon Press
McCabe D.P., Castel A.D. 2008. 'Seeing is believing: the effect of brain images on judgments of scientific reasoning'. *Cognition* 107, 343–52
Margolis, J. 1976. 'The concept of disease'. *Journal of Medicine and Philosophy* 1, 238–55
Marinker, J.H. 1975. 'Why Make People Patients?'. *Journal of Medical Ethics* 1, 81–4
Nessa, J. & K. Malterud 1998. 'Feeling your large intestines a bit bound: clinical interaction – talk and gaze'. *Scand J Prim Health Care* 16, 211–5
Nordby, H. 2006. 'The analytic-synthetic distinction and conceptual analysis of basic health concepts'. *Medicine Health Care and Philosophy* 9, 169–180
Nordenfelt, L. 1987. *On the Nature of Health*. Dortrecht, Kluwer
Nordenfelt, L. 1994. 'On the Disease, Illness and Sickness Distinction: A Commentary on Andrew Twadle's System of Concepts'. Twaddle, A. & L. Nordenfelt eds.: *Disease, Illness and Sickness: Three Central Concepts in the Theory of Health*. Linköping, Linköping University Press (Studies on Health and Society 18), 19–36
Nordenfelt, L. & B.I.B Lindahl eds. 1984. *Health, disease and causal explanations in medicine*. Boston, Reidel
Nordenfelt, L. 2007. 'The concepts of health and illness revisited'. *Med Health Care Philos* 10, 5–10
Parsons, T. 1951. *The Social System*. London, Routledge & Kegan Paul

Parsons, T. 1958. 'Definitions of Health and Illness in the Light of American Values and Social Structure'. Jaco, E G ed.: *Patients, physicians and illness : sourcebook in behavioral science and medicine.* New York, Free Press, 165–187

Parsons, T. 1964. *Social Structure and Personality.* New York, Free Press

Pellegrino, E.D. & D.C. Thomasma 1981. *A Philosophical Basis of Medical Practice.* Oxford, Oxford University Press

Pellegrino, E.D. & D.C. Thomasma 1993. *The virtues in medical practice.* Oxford, Oxford University Press

Pörn, I. 1993. 'Health and Adaptedness'. *Theoetical Medicine* 14, 295–303

Rather, L.J. 1958.' Zur Philosophie der Begriffs "Krankheit"'. *Deutsche Medizinische Wochenschrift* 83, 2012–8

Reiser, S.J. 1978. *Medicine and the Reign of Technology.* New York, Cambridge University Press

Reznek, L. 1987. *The nature of disease.* New York, Routledge & Keagen Paul

Rothschuh, K. 1972. 'Der Krankheitsbegriff. (Was ist Krankheit?)'. *Hippokrates* 43, 3–17

Ryle, G. 1949. *The concept of mind.* London, Hutchinson

Räikkä, J. 1996. 'The social concept of disease'. *Theoretical Medicine* 17(4), 353–61

Sachs, L. 1988. *Medicinsk Antropologi.* Stockholm, Liber

Sade, R.M. 1995. 'A Theory of Health and Disease: The Objectivist-Subjectivist Dichotomy'. *Journal of Medicine and Philosophy* 20, 513–25

Scadding, J.G. 1967. *Sarcoidosis.* London, Eyre & Spottiswoode

Sundström, P. 1987. *Icons of Disease: a philosophical inquiry into the semantics, phenomenology and ontology of the clinical conceptions of disease.* Linköping, Linköping University Press

Temkin, O. 1963. 'The Scientific Approach to Disease: Specific Entity and Individual Sickness'. Crombie, A C ed.: *Scientific Change: Historical Studies in the Intellectual, Social and Technical Conditions for Scientific Discovery and Technical Invention from Antiquity to the Present.* New York, Basic Books, 629–47

Tranøy, K.E. 1967. 'Asymmetries in ethics'. *Inquiry* 10, 351–372

Tranøy, K.E. 1995a. 'Om helsebegreper og helsetjeneste: en meditasjon'. Klockars, K & B Österman eds.: *Begrepp om hälsa: filosofiska och etiska perspektiv på livskvalitet, hälsa och vård.* Stockholm, Liber Utbildning, 127–139

Trանøy, K.E. 1995b. 'Grunnleggende etiske prinsipper i helsetjenesten'. Liss, P.E. & B. Petersson eds.: *Helsosamma tankar*. Nora, Nya Doxa, 145–54

Turner, B.S. 1987. *Medical Power and Social Knowledge*. London, Sage Publications

Twaddle, A. 1968. *Influence and illness: definitions and definers of illness behavior among older males in Providence, Rhode Island*. Ph.D. Dissertation, Brown University

Twaddle, A. 1994a. 'Disease, illness and sickness revisited'. Twaddle, A & L Nordenfelt eds.: *Disease, Illness and Sickness: Three Central Concepts in the Theory of Health*. Linköping, Linköping University Press (Studies on Health and Society 18), 1–18

Twaddle, A. 1994b. 'Disease, Illness, Sickness and Health: A Response to Nordenfelt'. Twaddle, A. & L. Nordenfelt eds.: *Disease, Illness and Sickness: Three Central Concepts in the Theory of Health*. Linköping: Linköping University Press (Studies on Health and Society 18), 37–53

Twaddle, A. 1973. 'Illness and Deviance'. *Social Science and Medicine* 7, 751–62

Twaddle, A. 1974. 'The Concept of Health Status'. *Social Science and Medicine* 8, 29–38

Twaddle, A. 1979. *Sickness behavior and the sick role*. Boston, Hall

Twaddle, A. & L. Nordenfelt eds. 1994. *Disease, Illness and Sickness: Three Central Concepts in the Theory of Health*. Linköping: Linköping University Press (Studies on Health and Society 18)

Tyreman S. 2006. 'Causes of illness in clinical practice: a conceptual exploration'. *Med Health Care Philos* 9, 285–91

World Health Organization (1947). Preamble to the Constitution of the World Health Organization adopted by the International Health Conference, New York, 19–22 June 1946; signed on 22 July 1947 by the representatives of 61 States (Official Records of the World Health Organization, no. 2, p. 100); and entered into force on 7 April 1948.

Wittgenstein, L. 1953. *Philosophical Investigations*. Oxford, Blackwell

Yong, A. 1982. 'The Anthropologies of Illness and Sickness'. *Annual Revue of Anthropology* 11, 257–85

Chapter 3

On the dynamics of sickness in work absence

Bjørn Hofmann

Summary

Traditionally, sickness is conceived of as a social identity, by which others acknowledge an individual's health problems with reference to his or her social activity and which generates certain rights and duties. However, structural changes, such as increased individualization and fragmentation, have altered the social perspective on sickness. The importance of the 'acknowledgement by others', and hence the intersubjective and social basis of the sick role, appears to be changing. In societies with well-functioning social security systems, the individual perspective (of illness) has increased in importance for sick leave and thus for the conception of sickness itself. This transformation challenges the traditional distinctions between disease, illness, and sickness as well as those between sickness absence, leave, and absenteeism, and it calls for a reinvestigation of these concepts. This chapter will analyze the dynamics of the key concepts of disease, illness, and sickness (the DIS-framework) as well as those of sickness absence, leave, and absenteeism (the work absence, or WA, framework). It is argued that these conceptual frameworks may still be useful for analyzing and addressing issues of health-related work absence. However, they should not be applied statically and stagnantly but in a complex dynamic manner, in particular, acknowledging the many actors and influencing institutions. This obviously makes the analyses less easy and the interventions less simple; however, using a map that follows the details of the terrain may improve one's overall orientation.

Introduction

There is a rich tradition in the controversies over human ailment. What is disease? Does this person qualify as diseased? Are you healthy when no disease can be identified? Who is authorized to decide whether you are diseased or not? When are you so sick that you cannot work? The questions are numerous, the disputes are ferocious, and agreement is absent (Hofmann 2001). It has been argued that the distinctions, originally made in social sciences, between disease, illness, and sickness are fruitful in order to sort out confusing concepts and challenging situations (Parsons 1958; Young 1982; Twaddle 1981; 1994a; 1994b; Hofmann 2002a; chapter 2 above). *Disease* is characterized as events or conditions (occurrences) that health care professionals consider to be of disadvantage (pain, suffering etc) to the individual. *Illness* is characterized as the person's first order perceptions of health problems, and sickness describes the sick role people assume when they have a disease, i.e. a state of social dysfunction (Last 1983; Tellnes 1989).

Table 1: Characteristics of three perspectives of human ailment: disease, illness and sickness.

	Disease	**Illness**	**Sickness**
Sphere	Professional	Personal	Society
Objective	Localise, explain and classify phenomena in the pursue for treatment, palliation and care	Explain a disvalued experience to oneself and others	Entitle legal and economical rights (and duties)
Perspective	Objective	Subjective	Inter-subjective
Attributes	Physiological, bio-chemical, bio-molecular, (mental) events	Suffering (pain)	Social status
Altruistic approach	Cure	Care	Recourse allocation, justice, equality

It has been argued that the distinctions between *disease*, *illness*, and, *sickness* are only philosophically defensible within a holistic theory of health (Nordenfelt 1994). I have earlier argued that this is not so (Hofmann 2002a). The concepts *disease*, *illness*, and *sickness* can be philosophically defended, and they highlight different perspectives on human ailment which can explain many of the conceptual and normative challenges that we face in modern welfare states. Table 1 illustrates the different perspectives.

However, the distinctions between *disease*, *illness*, and *sickness* cannot address all conceptual and normative challenges regarding human ailment. The vast and vibrant debates on sickness absence illustrate this. It has been argued that health-related work absence is too high, too costly, and unacceptably increasing (Waddell et al. 2007). Against this, it has been claimed that there is no significant shift in work absence but rather in the way absences are measured and counted (Hensing et al. 1998). Thus, there is little consensus on the extent of work absence and on what measures are adequate to reduce it.

Furthermore, some people feel stigmatized and accused of laziness when absent from work, or they feel forced to go to work even if they are diseased (this is known as 'sickness presence'). Others feel they have the right to stay away from work for a certain amount of days every year as part of social welfare arrangements. Physicians feel squeezed by obligations to their patients and by their duties as gate keepers to control work absence. Government authorities and employers seem desperately in need of ways to handle work absence in order to uphold production and control costs. Hence, sickness absence raises significant challenges to individuals, employers, insurance companies, health care providers, and public authorities. The challenges are personal, economic, moral, legal, (health care) professional, organizational, and governmental. The distinctions between *disease*, *illness*, and *sickness* may not address these issues in a satisfactory manner.

Part of the bewilderment may be due to lack of conceptual clarity and consistency beyond the *disease*, *illness*, and *sickness* distinctions. Conceptual divisions between *sickness absence*, *leave*, and *absenteeism* have turned out to be useful (Tellnes 1989). *Sickness absence* is when absence from work is caused by disease or injury (certified by health care personnel, self-certified, or uncertified), while *leave* is permission to be absent from work due to social obligations, such as maternity leave, children's sickness, civic duties, or funerals, and *absenteeism* is an unexcused or unauthorized absence or a shirking of one's duty. Many of the public debates appear to be confused because they confound various phenomena and concepts.

However, the distinctions between *disease*, *illness*, and *sickness* as well as between *sickness absence*, *leave*, and *absenteeism*, do not eliminate all challenges. Who is to define or certify sickness absence? Is it the individual, the professional, the insurer, the employer or society at large? Is there too much sickness absence? What is the appropriate level? Who is to decide? These and similar questions cannot easily be answered within the frameworks of *disease, illness, and sickness* (DIS-framework) or of *sickness absence, leave*, and *absenteeism* (the work absence, or WA-framework).

The above discussion stresses the need to revisit these frameworks to see whether they can shed light on these challenges. As changes create new challenges in health care, more dynamic concepts of health and disease are needed (Bircher 2005). This chapter will investigate the DIS-framework but will start by reviewing the dynamics of the WA-framework.

Table 2: Various forms of work absence characterized by their causes, certifications, and tentative background attitudes. Elaborated from Tellnes 1989.

Phenomenon	(tentative) Cause	Certification	Attitudes altered by
Sickness absence	Unhealth (malady) • disease, • illness • injury • impairment • sickness (sick role)	• Employer • Health professional • Person himself	• Unemployment • Responsibility • Solidarity • General welfare • Character of work (demanding, risky)
Leave	Social obligation • Maternity leave • Children's sickness • Funeral • Civic duties	Certifiable, but not necessarily certified	Social status of • Children • Pregnancy • Death • Civic institutions
Absenteeism	Breaking social norms • Shirking • Laziness • Inertia	Not certifiable, but normally not sanctioned	• Responsibility • Solidarity • Sense of coherence • Participation • Contribution

Absence

The various kinds of absence are normally characterized by various descriptions, like those given above (see also Tellnes 1989). However, it may be more fruitful to analyze work absence in terms of causes, certifications, and background attitudes. Table 2 indicates how various forms of work absence are justified and certified, as well how they may be promoted by various attitudes. *Sickness absence* is characterized by adhering to norms of health behavior. *Leave* is typified by social obligations, i.e., following social norms, whereas *absenteeism* is characterized by breaking standard social norms but without direct sanctions.

Hence, if we want to reduce absenteeism, it is not necessarily a brilliant idea to restrict the classifications for sickness certification. If we want to promote familial and civic duties, we cannot expect to reduce *leave* to zero. Relevant analyses and fruitful measures depend on addressing the dynamics in the WA-framework. Figure 1 illustrates some of the dynamic elements.

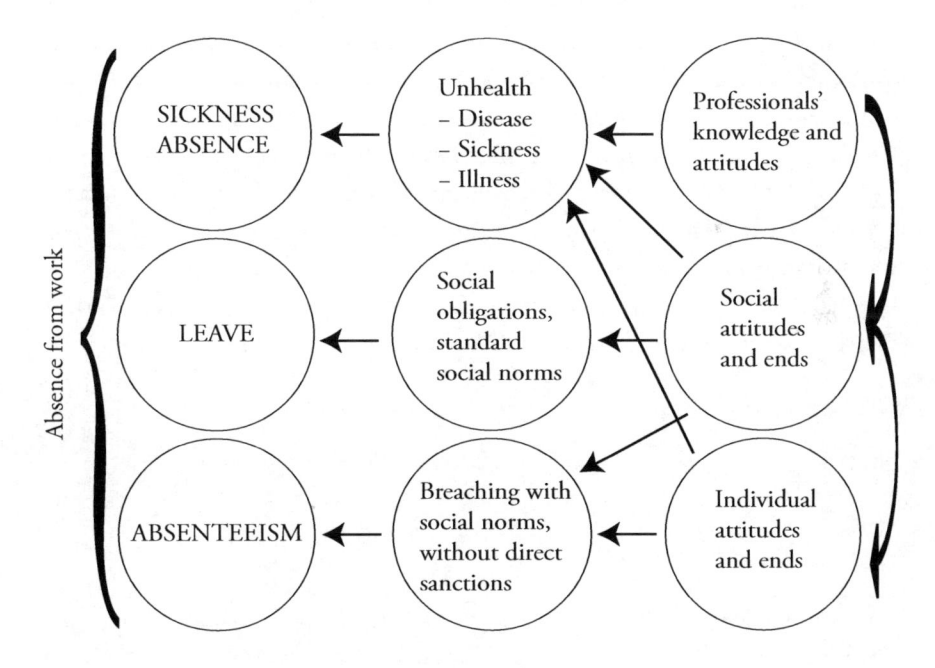

Figure 1: Sketch of the dynamic in work absence.

Could it be possible to reduce sickness absence by restricting self-certification? If sickness was a fixed concept and the DIS-framework was static, the answer would be 'yes', but this is exactly where health-related sickness absence challenges the DIS-framework. Sickness is not static. The conception of the sick role appears to be influenced by the levels of general welfare, unemployment, solidarity, and social responsibility. Restricted self-certification could reduce sickness absence in one situation but not in another, depending on various attitudes, for example.

Hence, a dynamic DIS-framework in general and a flexible sickness model in particular could be fruitful in order to address health-related work absence. That is, health-related work absence calls for a revision and refinement of the conceptual models of human ailment, which in turn can become fruitful on a more general level of health analysis.

On the dynamics of sickness

Although *disease*, *illness*, and *sickness* are characterized by a personal, a professional, and a social perspective respectively, they are not insulated or static. The concept of *illness* is influenced by both professional and social conceptions, just as that of *disease* is shaped by personal and social perspectives (Hofmann 2002a). The reason for this is that physicians are also sometimes patients and patient organizations promote particular conceptions of disease, e.g. to influence health insurers' coverage. Society actively funds research in particular areas, and health insurers engage in coverage discussions. As a result, it is reasonable to expect that the concept of sickness is influenced by personal and professional perspectives as well as by various social perspectives. Figure 2 sketches part of the dynamics among *disease*, *illness*, and *sickness*.[1]

---

[1] In health care systems like the Scandinavian one, health professionals are gate keepers and guardians of the sick role through sickness certificates. This means that the distinction and influence between *disease* and *sickness* is not necessarily mediated by external agents but can be 'internal' to a professional who plays more than one role.

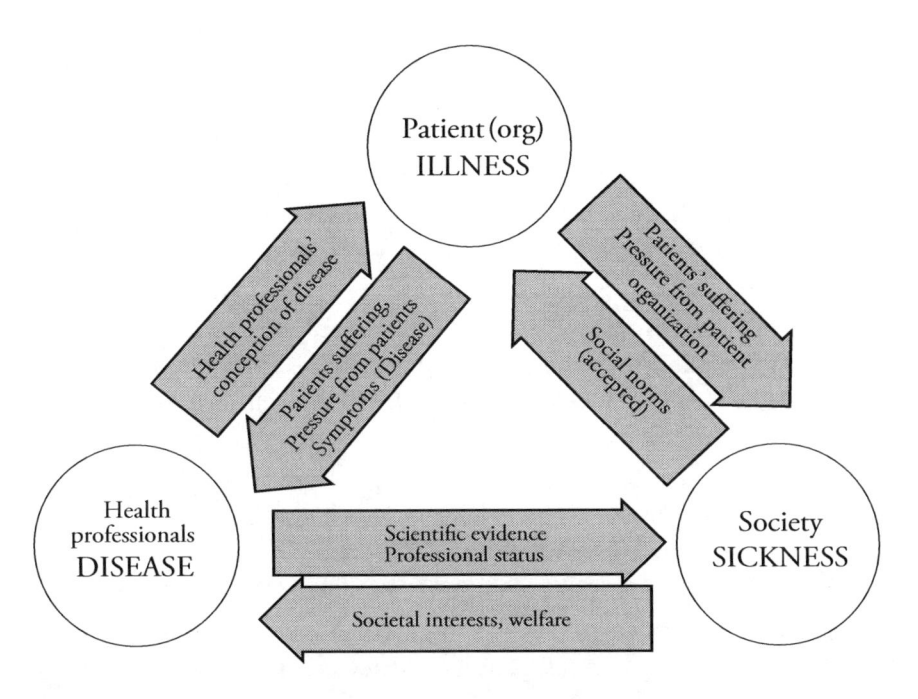

Figure 2: Sketch of the dynamic relationship between *disease, illness,* and *sickness.*

Although, *the sick role* may be influenced in a number of ways by numerous sources, suffice it here to point to some main dynamics.

Firstly, *sickness may be socially induced* in several ways, e.g. locally, on a group level, or in society at large (Virtanen et al. 2010). Whether pregnancy justifies sickness absence varies between countries and even within countries, as well as with time (Sydsjö et al. 1997).[2] The social conception and status of work, being active and coping, as well as the status of disease strongly influence what justifies or alters the sick role. The same goes for attitudes toward society, solidarity, and work as a social duty. Furthermore, the sense of coherence in people's lives as well as the feeling of uncanniness[3] may influence the sick role.

Thus, the attitudes towards health-related work absence may vary by workplace and over time. Sometimes, it is considered to be better for the workplace if the person is absent or recovers in absence, e.g., when it hampers production or prolongs the recovery time. Sickness may also be socially altered

---

[2] Note that pregnancy can, of course, also justify *leave*, but this is not the issue here.
[3] Heidegger uses the term 'Unheimlickeit', see Svenaeus (2000). So does Freud.

by society at large, e.g., through general conceptions of welfare. Widespread social attitudes like 'people in this condition should not (have to) work' also influence the sick role.

Second, *sickness may be instigated by health care professionals.* Health professionals' attitudes to particular conditions and their status may alter *the sick role*. For example, physicians' attitudes towards chronic fatigue syndrome (CFS) and obesity have changed significantly with professional attention and research findings. Health professionals may also respond to health-infringing working conditions, such as high work load, work place conflicts, and media pressure, and by altering health certification practices.[4] On the other hand, health professionals may restrict the sick role through their sickness certificate practices.

Third, sickness may also be instilled through personal attitudes. Shirking duties, laziness, and inertia are generally not acceptable, but they are implicitly accepted through a lack of direct response and reaction. Absenteeism breaks with formal norms but is oftentimes not sanctioned. The reasons for a lack of reaction may be manifold: the borders, delimitations, and definitions may be unclear, it may be unpleasant to sanction, or there may be an overly naïve social attitude.[5] The borders of sanction may be challenged, moved, and broken by individuals in relation to their (local) normative system. It is worth noting that the reactions and sanctions relevant for absenteeism stem from the person's social milieu and not primarily from health care professionals. Hence, more restrictive health certificate practices may have little direct influence on absenteeism.

Figure 3 summarizes the dynamics of the sickness concept discussed in this section.[6]

---

[4] For example, in Norway, the Stavanger bishop Baasland argued in a newspaper interview that he felt very fine, but, under the given circumstances (being personally bankrupt because he was cheated by his son), his doctor recommended him to accept sickness absence. 'I am healthy, but in the given situation my doctor recommended me to take sick leave until September' (Stokke 2008).

[5] The Norwegian language has a special word for this, 'snillisme', which means a naïve kindness, with often counterproductive effects.

[6] Other structural aspects, such as gender differences in occupational life (Laaksonen et al. 2010), may also play a role in the conception of sickness.

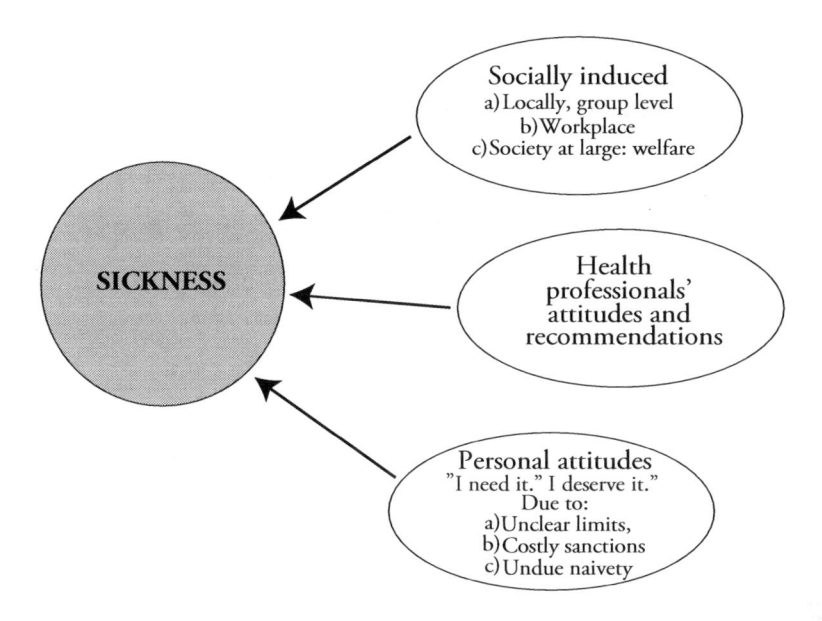

Figure 3: One perspective on the dynamics of sickness.

As we have seen, social attitudes, professional conceptions, and personal attitudes influence the sick role and what may be accepted as sickness leave. Put differently, the *zeitgeist* shapes *sickness*. Analyzing the factors influencing the sick role may be as fruitful in assessing sickness absence as counting sickness certificates. Further, such analysis is necessary in order to give direction and meaning to the counting exercise. Indeed, the analysis may indicate relevant measures for altering sickness absence that otherwise might be ignored. Trying to regulate personal attitudes through health care professionals' certificate practice may be as inappropriate as trying to adjust health professionals' conceptions of disease status and work ability through general social campaigns.

Agents of sickness ascription

Who, then, is to define sickness? Who should have the final say with regard to the sick role? As clear and relevant as these questions are, the answers are normally various and vague. One reason for this is the diversity of agents and institutions inducing and influencing the sick role. Some of these are illustrated in Figure 4.

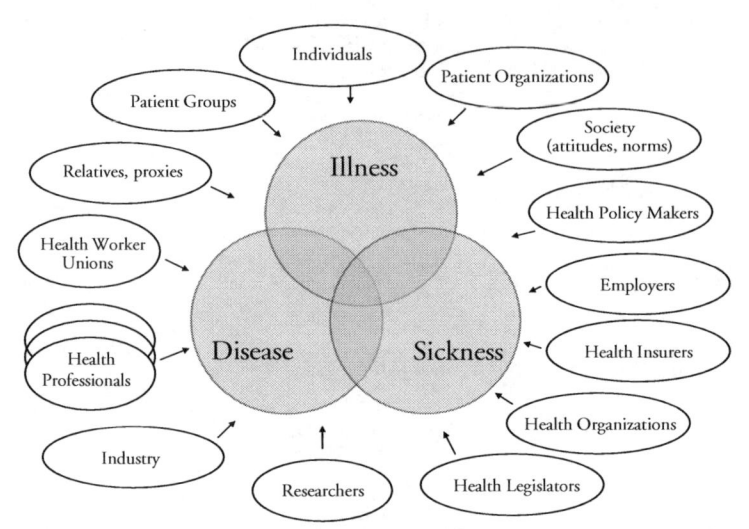

Figure 4: Overview of some of the actors influencing the conception of sickness as well as of disease and illness.

A detailed discussion of the agents' and institutions' various influences on *sickness* is beyond the scope of this chapter. Here, the discussion will be limited to the crucial question of who is to certify or attest sickness absence.

Although sickness certification has been widely delegated to physicians, there are several alternative trends, which are relevant for the development of the sick role. First, other health professionals have obtained the rights to certify sickness absence, for example, occupational physicians, physiotherapists, manual therapists, community psychiatric nurses, occupational therapists, and chiropractors (Whitacker 2001). This can expand the number of certification categories and certification practices.

Second, poor sickness absence management can result in long-term unemployment and influence health and well-being (Acheson 1998). It is strongly indicated that general practitioners do not readily engage in vocational rehabilitation (Coole 2010), and it has become widely accepted that employers should take greater responsibility for the management of sickness absence (CBI 2001). Accordingly, it can be argued that employers should take a more active part in sickness absence certification.

Third, health professionals are split between the gate keeper role for society in assuring justice and controlling health care costs, on the one hand,

and the role as the patient's advocate in issues of personal health, on the other. Third-party agents with professional health care competence have been used to try to avoid this conflict of interest and ensure justice (Söderberg & Alexanderson 2005).

Fourth, patient organizations and patient interest groups engage in debates on disease categorization. The aim of these various groups is to get 'their condition' on the list of accepted disease entities appearing on sickness certificates. Furthermore, there is a general interest among employees to promote self-certification of sickness.[7]

Hence, the various agents may be engrossed in different aspects of sickness: the health care professionals are preoccupied with sickness certification on basis of conceptions and classifications of disease, employers are preoccupied with sickness from the perspective of production loss and costs, while health care providers, authorities, and private insurers are engrossed by controlling sickness benefits, resource allocation, and cost containment. Additionally, patient and patient organizations are geared towards providing sickness benefits through relevant and liberal disease categories.

It is quite clear that these perspectives are not easily integrated. Ignoring the agents, institutions, and their interests can result in erroneous conceptions of sickness and misplaced measures to regulate sickness absence. Furthermore, highlighting the many agents influencing basic concepts in health care illustrates the complexity of the subject matter.

Sickness, identity, sin, and honor

One aspect of sickness that emerges from this analysis, one that appears to have been partly ignored in the literature, is the importance of one's self-conception for *sickness* and vice versa. It is well known that various diseases have different prestige among health care professionals (Album & Westin 2008). In general, different diseases give different social standing (Hofmann 2008). Having myocardial infarction (MI) has a different reputation than having fibrymyalgia or myalgic encephalopathy. This is important for the concept of

---

[7] It is worth noting that self-certification is not restricted to sickness but may include leave and other causes of absence than sickness. The vagueness of the concept of self-certification appears to result in much debate and confusion.

sickness. A hard working businessman getting MI more typically satisfies the sick role than, say, a part time worker with fibromyalgia.[8]

Although the medieval conception of disease as sin was abandoned long ago, diseases have normative connotations, which can still be recognized in the conception of *sickness*. The social aspects of *disease* categories are clearly reflected in the conceptions of *sickness*.

Diseases also invoke social identity. Some people insist on having certain diseases. It provides social identity and group belonging (Hofmann 2002b). On the other hand, some people take pride in not being sick, i.e. not being absent from work (Aronsson et al. 2005). Further, being sick can undermine the standing and identity of a professional. Think of a seasick boat crew member. The professional suitability of such a person may well be questioned if he or she gets repeatedly seasick. Furthermore, sickness absence can itself have negative health effects (Vingård Alexanderson & Norlund 2004).

The point is that *sickness* is related to personal identity and self-conception (through the social aspects of disease categories) in several ways. Influencing conceptions and behaviors relating to sickness cannot be accomplished through simple interventions. In particular, superficially addressing absenteeism through public campaigns and debates on health-related work absence may be counterproductive, if vulnerable persons who associate their sickness with (social) sin feel even worse and absentees who are immune to deontological demands for work participation remain unaffected.

Subjective sickness and objective absence?

Where then, does this leave us? The above analysis clearly shows the complexity of sickness and sickness absence. It illustrates how the WA-framework and the DIS-framework are useful for understanding and addressing issues of health-related work absence. However, it also shows that these frameworks have to be refined, elaborated, and enhanced in order to address important issues with regard to sickness absence. In particular, the WA- and DIS- frameworks need to integrate important dynamic aspects, which are often ignored in their static presentations.

---

[8] Even more, the businessman may be said to constitute a kind of prototype in the conception of sickness (Lakoff & Johnsen 1980).

Figure 5 tries to sum up some of the dynamic factors that are discussed in this chapter.

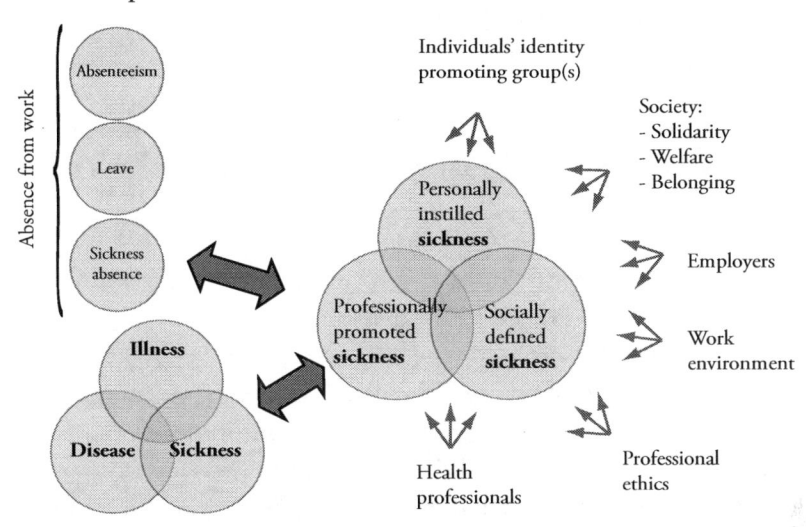

Figure 5: Summary of the dynamics of *sickness* highlighted through the combination of the *work absence* (WA) framework and the *disease, illness, and sickness* (DIS) framework.

The concept of *sickness* as an intersubjective conception of human ailment needs to be revised. The same goes for that of *disease* as an exclusively professional perspective and *illness* as a purely personal outlook on human ailment. It follows from the analysis that *sickness*, which has been the main focus of this chapter, is strongly influenced by professional attitudes and conceptions, not only among health care professionals but also among employers, colleagues, and those in one's own profession. Furthermore, *sickness* is also affected by personal preferences and individual conceptions of work, duty, belonging, group identity, self esteem, and solidarity. These conceptions do not emerge in a social vacuum but are constituted in a social sphere. However, how these conceptions are framed and formed differ significantly from one group to the next, and, even more interestingly, from one individual to another.[9] Hence,

---

[9] *Disease* is verified by the health care professionals, e.g., by diagnostic tests, and documented in the medical record. *Sickness* is also certified by health professionals, often based on disease verification. *Illness*, however, is neither verified nor certified, as it is basically a subjective concept. Although *illness* has been defined as an 'objective' measure, e.g., as an 'action failure' (Fulford 1993), it nevertheless depends on the individual's report.

the lesson learned is that *sickness* is also influenced by subjective and personal conceptions as well as by professional perspectives (Svensson et al. 2006). But if sickness can be subjective (to a certain extent), does this mean that sickness absence cannot be objective and impartially measured? The point here is that sickness has a series of premises, some subjective and others intersubjective, and that both measurements and measures to influence sickness absence have to take these premises into account. The concept of *sickness* without percepts is empty, and percepts without (the concept of) *sickness* are blind, to adapt Immanuel Kant's famous dictum.

In sum, the DIS-framework and the WA-framework are useful for analyzing and addressing issues of health-related work absence. However, they should not be applied statically and stagnantly (Niebrój 2006; Wikman and Marklund 2005; Bircher 2005) but in a complex dynamic manner, in particular, acknowledging the many actors and influencing institutions. This obviously makes the analyses less easy and the interventions less simple; however, having a map that follows the details of the terrain may be more successful in leading one to the desired destination.

Acknowledgements

This work is part of the project Social factors contributing to sickness absence which is funded by the Norwegian research council. I am most thankful to the project organizers, Rolf Rønning and Halvor Nordby and to the Norwegian research council.

References

Acheson, D. 1998. *Independent inquiry into inequalities in health report*. London, The Stationery Office

Album, D. & S. Westin 2008. 'Do diseases have a prestige hierarchy? A survey among physicians and medical students'. *Social Science and Medicine* no. 1, 182–188

Aronsson, G. & K. Gustafsson 2005. 'Sickness Presenteeism: Prevalence, Attendance-Pressure Factors, and an Outline of a Model for Research'. *Journal of Occupational and Environmental Medicine* no. 9, 958–966

Bircher, J. 2005. 'Towards a dynamic definition of health and disease'. *Medicine Health Care and Philosophy* no. 3, 335–41

Confederation of British Industry. *Their health in your hands: focus on occupational health partnerships.* London, CBI, September 2000

Coole C., P.J. Watson, & A. Drummond 2010. 'Work problems due to low back pain: what do GPs do? A questionnaire survey'. *Fam Pract* no. 1, 31–7

Hensing, G. et al. 1998. 'How to measure sickness absence? Literature review and suggestion of five basic measures'. *Scand J Soc Med* no. 2, 133–44

Hofmann, B. 2001. 'Complexity of the concept of disease as shown through rival theoretical frameworks'. *Theoretical Medicine and Bioethics* no. 3, 211–37

Hofmann, B. 2002a. 'On the triad disease, illness and sickness'. *Journal of Medicine and Philosophy* no. 6, 651–74

Hofmann, B. 2002b. 'Den perfekte sykdom'. *Utposten* no. 2, 22–26.

Hofmann, B. 2008. *Hva er sykdom*. Oslo, Gyldendal Akademisk

Jaco, E.G. ed.1958. *Patients, physicians and illness : sourcebook in behavioral science and medicine.* New York, Free Press

Lakoff, G. & M. Johnson 1980. *Metaphors We Live By*. Chicago, University of Chicago Press

Laaksonen, M. et al. 2010. 'Scand J Gender differences in sickness absence – the contribution of occupation and workplace'. *Work Environ Health* 2010 [Mar 9. Epub ahead of print]

Niebrój, L.T. 2006. 'Defining health/illness: societal and/or clinical medicine?' *J Physiol Pharmacol* Suppl no. 4, 251–62

Last, J.M. 1983. *A dictionary of epidemiology*. New York, Oxford University Press

Nordenfelt, L. 1994. 'On the Disease, Illness and Sickness Distinction: A Commentary on Andrew Twadle's System of Concepts'. Twaddle A & L Nordenfelt. *Disease, Illness and Sickness: Three Central Concepts in the Theory of Health*, 19–36

Parsons, T. 1958. 'Definitions of Health and Ilness in the Light of American Values and Social Structure'. Jaco, E.G. ed.: *Patients, physicians and illness : sourcebook in behavioral science and medicine.* NY, Free Press

Stokke, O. 2008. 'Biskop begjært konkurs'. *Aftenposten* 20.08. http://www.aftenposten.no/nyheter/iriks/article2604660.ece (Accessed 01.10.2010)

Svenaeus, F. 2006. *The Hermeneutics of Medicine and the Phenomenology of Health: Steps Towards a Philosophy of Medical Practice.* Dordrecht, Kluwer Academic Publishers

Svensson, T., U. Müssener & K. Alexanderson 2006. 'Pride, empowerment, and return to work: On the significance of promoting positive social emotions among sickness absentees'. *Work* no. 1, 57–65

Sydsjö, A., G. Sydsjö & B. Kjessler 1997. 'Sick leave and social benefits during pregnancy – a Swedish-Norwegian comparison'. *Acta Obstet Gynecol Scand* no. 8, 748–54

Söderberg, E. & K. Alexanderson 2005. 'Gatekeepers in sickness insurance: a systematic review of the literature on practices of social insurance officers'. *Health Soc Care Community* no. 3, 211–23

Tellnes, G. 1989. 'Sickness certification in general practice: a review'. *Fam Pract* no. 1, 58–65

Twaddle, A. & L. Nordenfelt eds. 1994. *Disease, Illness and Sickness: Three Central Concepts in the Theory of Health*. Linköping, Studies on Health and Society

Twaddle, A.C. 1981. *Sickness behavior and the sick role*. Cambridge MA, Schenkman

Twaddle, A. 1994a. 'Disease, illness and sickness revisited'. Twaddle, A. & L. Nordenfelt: *Disease, Illness and Sickness: Three Central Concepts in the Theory of Health*, 1–18

Twaddle, A. 1994b. 'Disease, Illness, Sickness and Health: A Response to Nordenfelt'. Twaddle, A & L Nordenfelt. *Disease, Illness and Sickness: Three Central Concepts in the Theory of Health*, 37–53

Vingård, E., K. Alexanderson & A. Norlund (Swedish Council on Technology Assessment in Health Care) 2004. 'Consequences of being on sick leave'. *Scand J Public Health* Suppl63, 207–15

Virtanen, P., Vahtera J., Nygård C.H. 2010. 'Locality differences of sickness absence in the context of health and social conditions of the inhabitants'. *Scand J Public Health*. [Mar 12. Epub ahead of print]

Waddell, G., K. Burton & M. Aylward 2007. 'Work and common health problems'. *J Insur Med* 2007, no. 2, 109–20

Whittaker, S. 2001. 'The management of sickness absence'. *Occup Environ Med* 58, 420–424

Wikman, A., S. Marklund & K. Alexanderson 2005. 'Illness, disease, and sickness absence: an empirical test of differences between concepts of ill health'. *J Epidemiol Community Health* no. 6, 450–4

Yong, A. 1982. 'The Anthropologies of Illness and Sickness'. *Annual Revue of Anthropology* 11, 257–85.

Chapter 4

Sickness absence as a social construction: A theoretical perspective

Rolf Rønning

Summary

The authors of this book are interested in how social factors influence experiences of illness, of sickness absence, and of exclusion. Different theoretical perspectives can be used to understand the social processes. In this chapter, I will outline a moderate social constructionist framework. Viewing sickness and sickness absence as social constructions may be an important supplement to the dominant bio-medical model. Within a social constructionist model, the expansion of diagnoses and the growth in sickness absence can be seen as mechanisms for social control, whereby medicine has an important function in controlling deviance in modern societies.

Background

The high rate of sickness absence is seen as a serious problem for public authorities in many countries, both because of the cost of the sickness benefits and because of lost work days. Many strategies are used to reduce sickness absence. The choice of strategy depends on how the phenomenon of sickness absence is understood and interpreted. A bio-medical model is still dominant, which means that a medical doctor is required to examine and to certify that a person has a disease with a diagnosis that qualifies for sickness absence. It may be a problem that the rules for sickness benefits in many countries are based on an evaluation of the person's ability to work, not on the diagnosis, but doctors nevertheless are accepted as the best gatekeepers to the given support.

Social factors are recognised as important, but not formally accepted in this system. However, in the scientific discussions as well as in medical practice, the influence of social factors has been accepted for decades. The growth and acceptance of the disciplines of medical sociology and social medicine can be seen as a symbol of this development.

The aim of this chapter is to figure out a theoretical model which portrays sickness and sickness absence as part of the social interaction in society. Using a moderate social constructionist perspective allow us to see the expansion of diagnoses and the increase in sickness absence as part of the social control of deviance in society. While formal control of deviance traditionally has been conducted by the Church or the state, medicine has authoritative standing in modern societies and can be an important agent for controlling deviance.

The sick role as deviant behaviour

There are different perspectives for understanding health and illness. A biomedical perspective sees people as natural entities and tries both to find exact indicators for different diagnoses and to draw objective conclusions. By contrast, a socio-cultural perspective focuses on people as cultural and social beings. Employing this perspective, we shall not try to draw objective conclusions but instead attempt to understand how people interpret themselves and their situations. The knowledge we can present is 'the social construction of reality'.

Berger & Luckmann (1996) see this process of social construction as consisting of different stages. In the first stage people construct a cultural product, for instance, the idea that homosexuality is a disease, or that strange behaviour is caused by mental illness. 'Objectivation' occurs when these cultural products take on an objective reality of their own and are viewed as part of an objective reality that is independent of the creators. 'Internalisation' happens when people learn about these supposedly 'objective realities' through socialisation. The 'realities' are then part of the taken-for-granted knowledge and vocabulary of a society. The Thomas theorem (Thomas & Thomas 1928,

572) fits into this perspective: 'If men define situations as real, they are real in their consequences'.

'Realities' in this sense are constantly being constructed and deconstructed. This process can be seen as part of the struggle between conflicting interests in the society, whereby the dominant groups force their understanding upon the subordinate groups. A Marxist might say that the dominant thoughts are the thoughts of the dominant groups. Humans are both natural and cultural and thus do not permit of a reduction to the former (Skjervheim 2002). Sickness and sickness absence can therefore be seen as part of the social interaction in society and the struggle between conflicting interests.

In one of his most influential writings, Parsons (1951) interpreted illness as a special type of deviant behaviour. To be ill is to perform a social role, and a sick person becomes exempt from the performance of certain normal social obligations. A diagnosis defines some of the expectations that attend the sick role, and we can view these expectations as moderating the relationship between the performer in the sick role and the social environment. The sick person is expected to behave in a special manner and to assist the process of recovery in order that the person can resume being a full member of the society. She is not responsible for her condition and cannot be expected to recover by an act of will (Conrad & Schneider 1992).

Illness is one of few accepted deviations in our society (Johannisson 2003). Parsons (1951) pointed out that both crime and illness dispose one to deviant behaviour and that they are both violations of norms that can be disruptive of social life, though the attributions of cause are different. If we consider deviance as intended or wilful, it tends to be defined as a crime, but if it is seen as unintended, it tends to be defined as an illness (Aubert & Messinger 1958). Since crime and illness are both designations of deviance, it becomes necessary to distinguish between the two, especially with reference to appropriate mechanisms of social control. It is in this context that Parsons developed his notion of 'the sick role' (Conrad & Schneider 1992).

Social control and deviance

In all societies, we find mechanisms for regulating individuals' behaviour. Some forms of behaviour are accepted, and some are not. Social control concerns how people define and respond to deviant behaviour (Horwitz 1990).

The norms for right and wrong may vary from one society to another, and they may vary over time. Some norms seem to be close to universal, as the norms prohibiting murder. But we can find exceptions even to this, like so-called 'honour killing'. Some behaviour is punished in some societies, like a woman walking alone in the streets, but is 'normal' in others. Social controls are attempts to influence deviance and conformity, and it is purposive actions (Horwitz 1990). Social control operates on both informal and formal levels. In textbooks about the developments of society, it is common to describe the developments in social control as evolving from the local and interpersonal level with informal sanctions to the societal and national level, with formalised mechanisms of social control. These latter mechanisms are usually state-run and performed by staff responsible for laws and regulations, like the police and the courts. Institutions such as education, welfare, the mass media, and medicine also have a role in the social control of deviance. Control can go hand in hand with help and support. Infants are controlled by being required to take vaccines at public health offices. Mothers get assistance, but the public authorities control the children's situation at the same time.

In complex societies, we find different styles of social control. Horwitz (1990) differentiates between a penal, a compensatory, a conciliatory, and a therapeutic style. On a penal model, punishment is the solution. On the compensatory model, payments are the solution, and people who have offended should pay those who have been offended. A conciliatory model is employed if there is close relation between the involved actors (as, for example, in a marriage), in which case negotiation is the solution. On a therapeutic model, the problem is the person's behaviour, and the solution is treatment of the individual.

In everyday life, informal social control may be the most common. Through our socialization into the society, we have internalised many norms about appropriate behaviour. Through interaction with other people, we are both subject to and performers of relational controls. Informal control takes many different forms in different settings, and we find both positive and negative sanctions (smiles, dirty looks, ridicules, harassment, etc.). In relation to the sick role, formal control is conducted through a medical doctor and the welfare system responsible for economical support, while informal control is exercised by colleagues, neighbours, and family members.

Deviance is a universal phenomenon. In this sense, deviance is 'normal' in society (Durkheim 1895/1938) and has a social definition (and function). Social groups make rules and enforce their definitions on members through judgments and social sanctions. The definition of deviance is a question of power. Some groups are able to define behaviour they do not like or accept as deviance. Through history, we have seen different dominating agents of social control in this sense. The church has been such an agent, for example, in the Middle Age when women were accused of witchcraft for different reasons and executed. In more secular societies, the church and the religious gate-keepers (i.e. priests and bishops) have lost most of their influence. However, the religious gate-keepers are still important in some predominantly Muslim countries, where they have the authority to give the right interpretation of the Koran. The state is important and uses legal control as its main instrument of control. Law can be seen as the creation and interpretation of specialised rules in a politically organised society, and these rules are formulated and administrated within a structure of interests (Quinney 1969). The definition of a problem is connected to the administration of it; we decide who possesses the problem and who is responsible for handling it. Drunk driving can thus be seen both as a social and a traffic problem (Gusfield 1975).

In our 'modern' societies, rational thinking and science are important in deciding right or wrong. We want statements to be supported by evidence. In such societies, medicine is used as an important agent in controlling deviance (Conrad & Schneider 1992; Conrad 2007). An interactionist approach to deviance would see medicine as a controlling agent and as relative to the social processes in society. By contrast, supporters of the positivist approach would reject this relativistic perspective. Instead, they would insist that deviance is real, and that it exists in the objective experiences both of the people who commit deviant acts and of those who respond to them. In discussing illness as deviant behaviour, we find both approaches to deviance. From our interactionist point of view, deviance is relative. Homosexuality has been treated both as a sin and a disease.

In our interactionist perspective, deviance is a socially defined and a socially ascribed condition. To be 'deviant' is status which is given by somebody. Different societal groups can define different phenomena as deviant or as social problems, and they may see each others' behaviour as deviant. But only powerful groups can impose their standards on society. Societies can be seen as having 'hierarchies of creditability' (Becker 1967). Medical associations and institutions usually have a high standing in such hierarchies. The authorities in a society draw attention to the deviant and regulate how the society should react in order to maintain social control. To solve the problems of deviance, it becomes important to find the causes of the behaviour and treat them in an appropriate way. If a problem is defined as a medical problem, the connection between diagnosis and cure is especially close.

The interactionist perspective focuses attention on the societal reactions to the process of labelling behaviour as deviant (Schur 1971). This is a process of collective rule-making, and here we find what Becker (1973) calls 'moral entrepreneurs', groups that lobby for the creation of social rules. In Becker's study, the Marijuana Act of 1937 rendered the sale and use of marijuana deviant. If we interpret moral entrepreneurs in a narrow sense, their aim was to make the use of marijuana a sin that should be punished. A recent example of moral entrepreneurship in Norway is the campaign that succeeded in making smoking in public places illegal and deviant.

When the goal is to define something as a medical problem that needs to be cured, we could talk about 'medical entrepreneurs'. Deviance is a product of enterprise. Moral entrepreneurs and other proponents of deviance definitions can operate in any social system with the power to impose definitions of deviance on its members (e.g., school, factories, etc.). But in modern society, only law and medicine have the legitimacy to construct and promote deviance categories with wide-ranging application. Within medicine, this power even transcends social and national boundaries. The labelling of a disease or an illness, the medical designation for deviance, is usually considered to have universal application (Conrad & Schneider 1992). This is because they are supposed to use objective criteria. In the next section, we will discuss in more detail the role of medicine in performing social control.

The medicalisation of society

Zola (1972) defined 'medicalisation' as a process whereby an increasing number of problems in everyday life are explained using a medical model and treated with medical instruments. Similarly, Ivan Illich (1976) worried about the expansion of the jurisdiction of the medical profession and 'the medicalisation of life' whereby many problems that formerly were not defined as medical became treated as such. For every new diagnosis, the space for 'normal' behaviour is reduced, and people lose control over their everyday life.

It is important to stress that the whole process of establishing a new diagnosis and a new disease is social, and those with the power to define the problem play decisive roles (Spector & Kitsuse 1977). The 'naming' has important political implications for the ownership of the problem and for the deviants (Goode 1969). Without a name, the illness is 'homeless'. An illness becomes 'real' when there is agreement about how to recognise it, how to confirm it, and how to name it. The acceptance has consequences for the way people with the diagnoses think of their illnesses and how other people think about them (Johannisson 2006). Diagnoses are interactive categories; people start to think, feel, and behave depending on the ascribed categories (Hacking 1998).

A diagnosis is not, however, a sufficient condition for defining a phenomenon as a disease. Kleptomania is a diagnosis, but it is still not accepted as a disease (Szasz 2007). There are several reasons for making diagnoses. There can be scientific reasons, including a wish to identify affected organs and the cause of an illness; professional reasons, for example, a desire to expand one's own territory of expertise; legal reasons, like justifying sanctions against special groups; and political reasons, like those related to the provision of funds for research and treatment (Szasz 2007).

The Diagnostic and Statistical Manual (DSM), used for the categorisation of diseases in the US, contained 106 diagnoses in 1952, and the number grew to almost 300 in the 1994 edition (Mayes & Horwitz 2005). Brante (2006) mentions, in his critique of DSM, several types of diagnoses without basis in scientific progress: committee diagnoses, absurd diagnoses, cultural-related diagnoses, moralistic diagnoses, *ad hoc* diagnoses, and inductively constructed diagnoses. Using examples from each group, he argues against the unreasonable growth in non-scientific diagnoses.

It may be useful to see the phenomenon of medicalisation as a matter of degrees, rather than an either-or situation (Conrad 1992). Disease has been defined as 'a specific destructive process in an organism, with specific causes and specific symptoms' (Webster's New Ideal Dictionary). This definition is clearly within a positivistic tradition and indicates that a disease may be caused by something from outside the body (e.g., a virus) invading it. Freidson (1970, 252) states that medicine is oriented toward seeking out and finding illness, 'which is to say that it seeks to create social meanings of illness where that meaning was lacking before'. He claims that medicine plays the role of a moral entrepreneur.

Illness can be defined as the state of being sick (Conrad & Schneider 1992) and linked to the sick person's experience (see chapter 2 and 6). Modern medicine is connected to the progress of the health situation in society. The successful elimination of many infectious diseases can be seen as a symbol of this progress, together with the advances in heart and brain surgery. According to McKeown (1979) and others, however, medicine did not play an important role in the elimination of infectious diseases. Improved housing and sanitary conditions were much more important. Even so, medicine has a powerful position in our societies, and it is employed in order to solve new problems that are identified as deviant. We all need, or may need, the assistance and knowledge of the medical hierarchy, and this gives them monopolistic power. In the United States, the medical hierarchy has been criticised for exploiting this situation. In Scandinavia, by contrast, the medical staff is seen as part of the welfare state, and medical power is executed through other professional groups, like nurses, physiotherapists, etc.; less attention is thus given to pure medical power (Riska 2003).

Our definitions of deviance are based on an understanding of what is normal. A medicalisation of a problem starts when some authorities define some deviations from the norm as problematic or unacceptable. This is obvious a question of power, like when the rulers in the Soviet Union defined their critics as mentally ill and placed them in psychiatric institutions. In the US, a well-known physician introduced 'drapetomia', a disease whose main symptom was being a slave who runs away from a plantation (Cartwright 1851).

With varying degrees of tolerance, different forms of deviant behaviour have been treated as insanity. In order for a case of non-acceptable deviance to be medicalised, a theory is needed about the connection between the deviance and some medical and biological factors. Alternatively, the medical profession might claim it is able to solve the problem, for example, in the case of obesity, for which surgery is now used. There is an interesting question concerning when and for whom being overweight is a problem. In societies in which the majority are overweight, the thin people are deviants, like, for example, amongst the Papago Indians of Americas Southwest (Conrad & Schneider 1992). Labelling a situation or behaviour dysfunctional presupposes a standard of what is normal or well-functioning. Today, alcoholism is treated as a disease in hospitals, though many people still see it as a lack of moral strength. Disruptive behaviour in school can now be seen as a disease and cured with medicine, e.g., Ritalin. There are many different explanations of the expansion of ADHD diagnoses, and not all of them are medical (Brante 2006). We can see a development from badness to sickness, and the adoption of a medical model for a number of categories of deviant behaviour (Conrad & Schneider 1992).

In addition to the bio-medical model, psychotherapy has been established as a scientific medical discipline, an establishment which has been described as the 'triumph of the therapeutic' (Rieff 1966). Szasz (2007) has argued for a strong distinction between body-bounded diseases and mental diseases, by claiming that disease or illness only can affect the body. Brain diseases may change the function of the brain and cause severe problems, but the concept of 'mental disease' is a metaphor because it is not connected to any part of the body. 'Mental misbehaviour' is behaviour, not a disease, and the treatment will be society's strategic reaction to the deviant behaviour. Szasz' position is controversial, but it reminds us of the close connection between diagnoses and social control. Perhaps we have already seen the golden age of therapy; Conrad (2007) states that chemical treatments today seem to substitute for different forms of therapeutic intervention.

In their seminal book from 1980, reprinted in 1992, Conrad and Schneider saw the medical hierarchy (including medical doctors, their associations, universities, and research institutes) as the main drivers in the medicalisation of society, in combination with the authorities' need for social control of deviance. In a recent update, Conrad (2007) sees a change in this process with new actors and interactions. But the process of medicalisation of society has continued and even escalated, in the same direction: numerous studies have emphasized how medicalization has transformed the normal into the pathological and how medical ideologies, interventions, and therapies have reset and controlled the borders of acceptable behaviour, bodies, and states of being (Conrad 2007, 13).

He concludes that the key to medicalisation is still definition. Some statistics can illustrate the expansion of medicine: the percentage of GNP spent on health care has increased from 4.5% in 1052 to 16% in 2006 in the US, and the number of physicians per 100 000 residents has increased from 148 in 1972 to 281 in 2003 (Conrad 2007). A much more visible driver in the medicalisation process today is the pharmaceutical industry. New developments in psychopharmacology, neuroscience, and genomics have increased the influence of these big firms. Some authors see the development as a 'biomedicalisation' (Clarke et al. 2003). In USA (and New Zealand), pharmaceutical firms have been allowed to advertise directly to the consumers (DTC). In 2004, 4.5 billion dollars were spent on advertising medications and focusing on the ills they are meant to treat (Conrad & Leiter 2005).

One important branch of expansion has been so-called 'off-label use'. This happens when a drug is used in areas and fields other than those for which it was developed. These extended applications are very profitable for the firms. This use of medicine has been labelled 'cosmetic psychofarmacology' (Vedamtam 2001, 1). For example, Paxil was developed for the depression market, but it was also advertised to cure 'social phobia', which was defined as 'fear of social and performance situations in which embarrassment may occur' (Conrad 2007, 17). Advertising, together with other changes in the society, has transformed patients into consumers, and consumers are important allies for the firms. The sale of antidepressants in Sweden is now seven times higher than it was in 1993, and 600 000 Swedes are either using, or have access to, these drugs daily (SOU 2009, 89). In the beginning of 2009, 176 000 Norwegians were treated with antidepressants.

Many forces contribute to the growing consumption of medicine. Sometimes public authorities, who often have to pay the bill, also function as drivers; for example, categorising the swine-flu as a pandemic generated enormous profits for the multinational medical corporations. The situation is undisputable positive for the corporations, and it may be positive for many of the users. However, off-label uses of medicines result in an unforeseen increase in use; a Swedish study concluded that three of four using antidepressants in a nursing home lacked diagnoses that could motivate such treatment (Ulfarvarson 2004). Another expansion of medicine is the effort to treat 'protodiseases' (Conrad 2007), for instance, symptoms such as high blood pressure or high cholesterol. These conditions are not diseases in themselves but are seen as worrying and treated with drugs. Human differences are transformed into pathologies, like differences in learning style, sexual desires, breast size, etc. (Conrad 2007).

Illich (1976) labelled the process of medicalisation as 'medical imperialism', but this phrase misses the collective actions that we now see in the field.

There is both a medicalisation from above and a medicalisation from below (Szasz 2007). The big corporations are now seen as the main drivers from above, together with public authorities and the medical profession. Some observers find this alliance to be so strong in the US and the forces of 'coercive paternalis' to be so dominating that they label the system 'pharmacracy' (Szasz 2007). The forces from below are consumers—both individuals and organised groups—and social movements. The right to be accepted as having a disease is important in our system, both because of the legitimation and the access to benefits, and because the society accepts individuals' situations as real and does not consider them to be fakers or 'imaginary invalids' (Molière).

Many groups of people have struggled hard to get their situation accepted as a disease; diffuse musculoskeletal diseases and burnout are two examples. Medicine may support these groups and then add more space to their professional domain. In this sense, medicine is an agent for what Habermas (1984) called the system's invasion of the life-world. However, the development is not unidirectional, and we also find a demedicalisation of phenomenon. This underlines the dynamic and contextual role of diagnosis. The treatment of homosexuality and masturbation are examples here; both used to be treated as sins and diseases.

There are some forces resisting the medicalisation of society; groups believing in alternative treatments are one example. But these groups are seldom very strong. In the US, the insurance companies restrict the number of problems that are covered, while in Norway and Sweden, we expect the state to play a similar role. The insurance companies may raise the premiums to cover new costs, but then they become more expensive. It may be more difficult for the state to legislate higher taxes to cover additional tasks.

The medicalisation of society has many positive aspects, not least for the 'deviants'. Medicalisation fits into a humanitarian trend in society. Alcoholics are no longer arrested, but instead they are treated and accepted. This may have caused more tolerant and less condemning attitudes towards them. Medicalisation also allows for an extension of the sick role to those labelled as deviants. This removes blame from the individual and absolves people of responsibility for their behaviour. The sick role allows for the 'conditional legitimation' of a certain amount of deviance, as long as the individual fulfils the obligations of the sick role (Conrad & Schneider 1992). The price is that the sick person has to confirm that the illness itself is an undesirable state, and she has to cooperate in order to recover as quickly as possible (Parsons 1972). A medical model will often offer the deviant an optimistic outcome; there is a cure that will help (Pitts 1968).

Medicalisation lends the prestige of the medical profession to the treatment of the deviants; it is better to be treated as a sick person than as a sinner. Medical control of deviance is often more flexible and efficient than judicial and legal controls. On the negative side, we have to mention the dislocation of responsibility and its separation from social action. Since medicine is supposed to be objective and value-free, the moral judgements may be hidden. Also, parts of our fate are left to experts. Medicine as a tool for social control will tend to treat both social and societal problems as individual ones. Medicine always tries to cure the individual, not the society. The depoliticization of deviant behaviour can be the result (as in the Soviet Union) (Conrad & Schneider 1992).

Bringing in a social and cultural perspective on sickness allows us to see other explanations than those brought forward by the dominating bio-medical model. By focusing on the medicalisation of society, we can see drivers influencing the rates of sickness in society other than the 'sick' persons. This is important for the discussion about sickness benefits, because solutions to the problem have to take into account the contributions of different drivers.

From sick to sickness absence and sickness benefits

As explained by Parson (1951), the sick role gives the person freedom from normal duties, if others can take care of them. If it is not obvious that the person is sick, or there may be some doubt about the diagnosis, then the willingness to take on the other's duties may be lower or non-existent. The medical doctors (GPs) are the gate-keepers to the 'freedom from duties' status. In the Scandinavian welfare states, this is an important function, because those certified as sick are entitled to benefits. While we normally have to work for our income, this situation allows us to receive money without working.

It is not obvious that the doctors should have this role as gatekeepers, because the connection between having a disease and being unable to work is not necessarily close. A broken leg is difficult for bicycle messenger, but not so difficult for an author. A decision about peoples' ability to work when they claim an illness can be complicated, and it must be based on an individual evaluation of the relation between the sick person and his or her tasks. But since the result is important both for the employer and the employee, decisions have to be taken by someone with mutually accepted authority. Since an examination of the health situation should be undertaken first, there is good reason to leave the whole certification process to the GPs and to the medical system generally. They have the necessary authority to be accepted by both parties. In this situation, the public authorities have been the drivers in the medicalisation process. But when exactness is wanting in the diagnosis of ill people, the uncertainty is much higher. Bureaucrats in the social security system may question the given diagnosis when people are declared unfit to work, and the social security system has its own medical expertise for control sickness absence certificates. That said, the main picture is that the medical system decides about the ability to work and distributes sickness benefits. Clinical examinations have been important administrative tools in the welfare state, and such examinations leave one with a false impression of objectivity (Stone 1984). We know that a given diagnosis may be wrong, insufficient, and/or based on subjective discretion. We also know that, as a rule, it is the individual that contacts a doctor, and, in most cases, their own opinion will be accepted by the doctor.

The relation between the doctor and the individual is important for the outcome of the process about sickness benefits. The relation between the individual and the rest of the society is also important. People create and are created by society (Berger & Luckmann 1966). We are both participants and spectators in society (Skjervheim 2002). We learn to know about ourselves through interactions with other members of the society. It is therefore also important to pay attention to how sick-leave identities are created as a function of the social interaction between those sick-listed and their social networks and to keep general attitudes towards sick-leave and sick-listed in society in mind. The sick-listed individuals may identify themselves with external attitudes to sickness. An individual's interpretations of the sick role and the reactions from the social surroundings may influence the recovery. It is important to know, therefore, the general attitudes towards sick leave and towards different diagnoses, what people on sick leave expect the reactions in their social network to be, and how they experience them. A person can have an illness without sickness absence and can conversely have sickness absence without having an illness (chapter 3, 6 above). Some social networks may be more willing to accept different forms of sick leave than others. The person's own capabilities and interpretation of the situation, along with the reactions from the network, may be important here. We can see this as a negotiating process (Strauss et al. 1997); the acceptance of the illness and the limits are constructed in the interaction between the individual and 'significant others', especially in situations with diffuse diagnoses. The society and our social networks both support us and execute social control. Different social actors have different interests, and the outcome is not a given. Being accepted as a sickness benefit recipient varies in different social settings, it varies over time, and it depends on what kind of diagnoses one gets. To understand the social situation for the sickness absentees, it is important to consider how identities are formed in interaction with other people. Of special interest to this study are attitudes to different kinds of mental diagnoses. We know from the literature that the label of mental illness is linked to an array of negative stereotypical traits, and that people with a mental diagnosis run the risk of being stigmatized (Corrigan & Lundin 2001; Scheff 1966). These groups are particularly subjected to shaming in the form of humiliation, belittling, and condescending and patronising treatment. Many people would regard them as being of lesser value. People with mental illness thus suffer the most from stigma.

Illness is a problem for the individual. If many people have health issues, it becomes a public problem. A few people being sickness absent does not constitute a public problem, but if many people are, then it becomes a public problem (Wright Mills 1959). When a problem is recognised as public, it gets public attention, and actors in the public debate will try to define the problem in their own way. If certain parties succeed in establishing a hegemonic discourse (Gramsci 1971), then they will have also garnered acceptance for their way of solving the problem. A dominating understanding will influence both people's own understanding of their problem and the reactions from society.

Sickness absence as a social phenomenon[1]

We do not have much knowledge about sickness absence as a social phenomenon, but there are some studies. In Sweden, sickness absence was established as a public problem at the end of the last century. A study of the public debates from 2000–2009 identifies two dominating discourses fighting for

---

[1] In this paragraph most of the references are taken from Starrin (2010).

the hegemony. The first discourse was concerned with the working conditions, claiming that more stress and growing psychosocial problems were the main factors. On this view, the employees were victims of a growing cruelty in the labour market. The labour unions were the main proponents of this discourse, and they dominated the media in 2000–2001. The other discourse was the 'over-consumption' discourse, which claimed that people used sickness absence as an income without have a disease or an illness. This view stressed that it was too easy to get the allowances and that they were too generous. This discourse started to get support from 2002, became strong 2003–2004, and has been hegemonic from 2005 (Johnsson 2010).

Palmehag (2007) has studied the media's coverage of sickness absence in the period from 1997–2006 and confirms Johnsson's picture. She analysed the content in five newspapers. During the first period, sickness absence was described as a symptom of other problems that had to be solved, for instance, poor working conditions. The absentees were victims of a bad situation, and they needed to get sympathy and support. One common explanation for the unpleasant situation was said to be job-closures following the economic crisis in 1990–1994. In the beginning of 1994, there was a shift in the debate. Less attention was given to the sickness absentees as victims. A new conception of them as people who chose to get sickness benefits without being 'really sick' was established. They were portrayed as people who preferred to stay out of the workforce with sickness benefits instead of accepting support as jobless and then having to meet demands for rehabilitation and moving (to new jobs). In the debate, people talked about withering norms, 'abuse' of rights, and cheating. The Swedes were said to be soft and naïve to let people on sick leave prolong their period. The refund level was too high and generous (Frykman & Hansen 2009).

Results from research projects performed by the Social insurance agency (Riksförsäkringsverket) gave support to statements about abuses of the system. They provided numeric evidence that people did misuse the system, and they documented cheating of the system. A journal (Svensk Näringsliv 2005) followed up these findings and published a report, wherein a majority of the respondents claimed that it was acceptable to ask for sickness benefits without having an illness (Modig & Boberg 2002). In the middle of the 1990s, Svallfors (1996) investigated the Swedish people's attitudes towards sickness absence. He found that 70% agreed with the statement: 'Many of the sickness absentees are not really sick'. More recently, TCO (a Swedish labour union) interviewed a group of personnel officers, and 56% confessed that they had negative or very negative attitudes toward hiring people who were on sickness absence in other organisations. 44% expressed negative attitudes towards hiring long-term unemployed (Rautio & Mörtvik 2005). These findings indicate scepticism about the abilities of people who are, or have recently been, out of the workforce.

People have different reasons to be on sick leave. In addition, diagnoses have different degrees of prestige among the caregivers. Hearth problems, leukaemia, and brain tumours have a high degree of prestige. Among the lowest ranked, one finds fibromyalgia, liver disease, and depression. This can indicate that diseases with diffuse causes and those that can be caused by a problematic way of living get little prestige (Album 1991; Album & Westin 2008). In a recent survey, Handisam (2010),[2] found that one in four Swedes preferred not to work with a person who had a mental disease, and one in five would not invite them home. This is in line with international studies, they conclude. As mentioned before, mental problems are the most frequent diagnoses for women on sick leave in Sweden.

Vidman (2009) concludes that many long-term sickness absentees experience that people in the environment seem to have doubts about their situation. When they are participating in recreational activities, other people seem especially apt to question both their sickness and their eagerness to recover. Some of the absentees react with isolation and withdraw from public arenas. Others try to ignore the reactions from the surroundings and try to live as normal a life as possible. Vidman's observations are contested by ethnologists Frykmans & Hansen's (2009) study. In two sparsely populated municipalities they investigated, people did not seem to withdraw from their normal social behaviour when they were on sick leave. Further, most people seemed to have a positive and relaxed attitude towards the absentees. Vidman concluded that sickness absence decreases people's self confidence. They feel that people gossip about and distrust them, and they always have to consider what to say and what to do. These feelings are not only subjective impressions; one of the informants was three times reported to the Social Security agency for cheating, and each times she proved to be innocent.

---

[2] Handisam is a cooperate organisation for the Swedish Association of the handicapped.

Conclusion

Viewing sickness as a socially constructed phenomenon may be a useful supplement to the dominant 'objective' medical model. For sickness absence, this may even more obvious. Public authorities have the power to define social deviations, and diagnoses of sickness can be used as a tool for social control. Many interest groups in the society work for the acceptance of new diagnoses and for a further medicalisation of society. The drivers are thus not only individuals who want to get money in an easy way, as suggested by the 'over-consumption' discourse.

The performance of the sick role for those receiving sickness benefits has to be done on a public stage for an audience in charge of the social control of deviants. The medical system is still the main gatekeeper, but other actors do not completely trust their control and may express their own opinions. Sickness absentees may then have to negotiate their own understanding of the illness in different arenas: at home, in the workplace, etc. The dominant understanding of the situation will influence both the absentees' interpretation of the situation and the reactions from the society. These reactions may vary over time, between different social groups, and depend on the diagnosis. Empirical studies are needed to give us a better understanding of this phenomenon.

References

Aubert, V. & Messinger, S.L. 1958. 'The criminal and the sick'. *Inquiry*, 137–160

Album, D. 1991. 'The prestige of diseases and medical specialities'. *Tidsskrift for den Norske Lægeforening*, 232–236

Album, D. & Westin, S. 2008. 'Do diseases have a prestige hierarchy? A survey among physicians and medical students'. *Social science and Medicine*, 182–188

Becker, H.S. 1967. 'Whose side are we on?' *Social Problems*, 239–471

Becker, H.S. 1973. *Outsiders*. New York, The Free Press

Berger, P.L. & T. Luckman 1966. *Den samfunnsskapte virkelighet*. Bergen, Fagbokforlaget

Brante, T. 2006. 'Den nya psykiatrin: exemplet ADHD'. Hallerstvedt, G. ed.: *Diagnosens makt*. Gøteborg, Daidalos

Cartwright, S.W. 1851. 'Report on the diseases and pecularities of the negro race'. *N O Medical Surg. Journal,* 691–715

Clarke, A. et al. 2003. 'Biomedicalization: Technoscientific Transformation of Health, Illness and U.S.Biomedicine'. *American Sociological Review,* 161–94

Conrad, P. & Schneider, J. 1992. *Deviance and the Medicalization of Society.* Philadelphia,Temple Press

Conrad, P. 1992. 'Medicalization and Social Control'. *Annual Review of Sociology,* 209–31

Conrad, P. & Leiter, V. 2005. 'From Lydia Pinkham to Queen Levitra: Direct- to-Consumer Advertising and Medicalization'. Paper presented at the meeting of the American Sociological Association, Philadelphia

Conrad, P. 2007. *The Medicalization of Society.* Baltimore. John Hopkins University Press

Corrigan, P.W. & Lundin R. 2001. *Don't call me nuts: Coping with the stigma of mental illness.* Tinley Park, IL, Recovery Press

Durkheim, E. 1938. *The rules of sociological method.* New York, The Free Press. First published in 1895

Freidson, E. 1970. *Profession of Medicine.* New York, Harper & Row Publishers

Frykman, J. & Hansen, K. 2009. *I Ohälsans tid.* Stockholm, Carlssons Bokförlag

Goode, E. 1969. 'Marihuana and the politics of Reality'. *Journal of Health and Social Behavior,* 83–94

Gusfield, J.R. 1975. 'Categories of ownership and responsibility in social issues: alcohol abuse and automobile use'. *Journal of Drug Issues,* 285–303

Gramsci, A. 1971. *Prison notebook.* London, Lawrence & Wishart

Hacking, I. 1998. *Mad Travellers: Reflections on the Reality of Transient Mental Illnesses.* London, Free Associations books

Horwitz, A. 1990. *The Logic of Social Control.* New York, Plenum Press

Illich, I. 1972. *The Medical Nemesis.* New York, Pantheon books

Johnson, B. 2010. *Kampen om sjukfrånvaron.* Lund, Arkiv förlag

Johannisson, K. 2006. 'Hur skapas en diagnos? Et historisk perspektiv'. Hallerstvedt, G. ed.: *Diagnosens makt.* Gøteborg, Daidalos

Mayes, R. & Horwitz, A. 2005. 'DSM –III and the Revolution in the Classfication of Mental Illness'. *Journal of the History of Behavior Sciences,* 249–268

McKeown, T. 1979. *The Role of Medicine*. Oxford, Basic Blackwell
Modig, A. & Boberg, K. 2002. 'Är det rätt att sjukskriva sig fast man inte är sjuk?' http://www.temo.se/uppload/334/22785r.pdf
Palmehag, A. 2007. *Från offer till attityd –en studie av hur sjukskrivningar beskrivits i svenske tidningar 1997–2006.* Lunds universitet, Arbeidsrapport
Parsons, T. 1951. 'Illness and the role of the Physician: A Sociological Perspective'. *American Journal of Orthopsychiatry*, 21 (3), 452–460
Pitts, J. 1968. 'Social control: the concept'. Sills, D. ed.: *International encyclopedia of social sciences*. New York, Macmillan
Quinney, R. A. 1969. 'A sociological theory of criminal law'. Quinney, R. ed.: *Crime and Justice in Society.* Boston, Little, Brown & co
Rautio, K. & Mörtvik, R. 2005. *Jakten på superarbetskraften.* Stockholm, TCO-rapport no. 16
Regeringens proposisjon 2007/08:136, 2008. *En reformerad sjukskrivningsprocess för ökad återgång i arbete*
Rieff, P. 1966. *Triumph of the Therapeutic.* New York, Harper & Row Publishers
Riska, E. 2003. 'Developments in Scandinavian and American medical sociology'. *Scandinavian Journal of Public Health*, 389–94
Scheff, T.J. 1966. *Being Mentally Ill III: A Sociological Theory.* Chicago Aldine
Schur, E.M. 1971. *Labeling Deviant Behavior.* New York, Harper & Row Publishers
Skjervheim, H. 2002. *Mennesket*. Oslo, Universitetsforlaget
SOU 2009:89 *Gränslandet mellom sjukdom ock arbete*
Spector, M. & Kitsuse, J. 1977. *Constructing Social problems.* Menlo Park, Cal., Benjamin Cummings Publishing Co
Starrin, B. 2010. *Sjukskriving och sjukfrånvaron som ett socialt fenomen.* Karlstads universitet. Arbetspapper 31.3.
Stone, D. 1984. *The Disabled State.* Philadelphia, Temple University Press
Strauss, A. et al. 1997. *Social Organization of Medical Work.* New Brunswick (US), Transaction books
Svallfors, S. 1996. *Välfärdens moraliska ekonomi – Välfärdsopinionen i 90-talets Sverige.* Umeå, Borea
Szasz, T. 2007. *The Medicalization of EveryDday Life.* Syracuse University Press
Thomas,W. & Thomas, D. 1928. *The Child in America.* Alfred Knoph

Ulfvarson, J. 2004. *Drug treatment of elderly.* Stockholm, Karolinska Institutet
Vendamtan, S. 2001. 'Drug Ads Hyping Anxiety Make Some Uneasy'. *Washington Post,* July 18
Vidman, Å. 2009. 'Långtidssjukskriving som en fråga om att bete sig rett'. In Sandvin, J. ed. *Arbete, sjukskriving och moral.* Lund, Studentlitteratur
Wright Mills, C. 1959. *The Sociological Imagination.* Oxford University Press
Zola, I.K. 1972. 'Medicine as an institution of social control'. *Sociological Review,* 487–504

Chapter 5

Aspects of sickness certification and work ability

Gunnar Tellnes

Summary

This chapter focuses on different phenomenon and tasks that general practitioners and other health personnel have to manage and be familiar with when they assess a person's capacity for work. Doctors' sickness certification practice, functional assessments, and work ability assessments, as well as occupational rehabilitation in the field of sickness absence, have been evaluated through different studies in Norway. Recent research indicates that multi-disciplinary occupational rehabilitation programs significantly improve perceived work ability when compared with treatment as usual. Beyond this, persons with illness and disease need inspiration and motivation to promote their health and to improve their capacity for work.

Introduction

One of the great challenges for persons certified sick due to chronic diseases concerns how they may return to work. Many research and rehabilitation efforts have been undertaken in Norway and other countries over the last 25 years to cut this 'Gordian knot', but so far the real solution is difficult to find. In spite of the increase in research on sickness absence during the last years, a review concluded that 'research on sickness absence and disability pension was found to be very undeveloped with regards to theories, methods, as well as concepts' (Alexanderson 2005). One of the challenges is also that the legislation and management of sickness absence across Europe and the rest of the world varies considerably, with, for example, different countries enforcing different periods of time available for self-cerification (Wynne-Jones et al. 2008). To establish and compare a baseline rate of sickness certification, as well as sickness absence, across countries, standardized reporting is needed. In addition, inter-doctor variation in sickness certification is also a challenge in this field of research and practice (Tellnes, Sandvik & Moum 1990. See also chapter 2 and 3).

The purpose of this chapter is to discuss aspects of sickness certification in Norway and its relation to function, work ability, occupational rehabilitation, and methods for returning to work. The main aim is to show that some recent studies in Norway imply that it is important to adopt a salutogenic approach to health and work ability. The literature on long-term sickness certification has traditionally focused on how it is possible to reduce health problems and make work-related arrangements in order to reduce sickness certification. The chapter supports the idea that the most important aim should be to promote health. In order to understand how we can achieve this aim, much more research with an alternative focus is needed (See more in Chapter 12).

Sickness certification and measurements used

Sickness certification data offer special statistical challenges. The great number and diversity of measurements used make it difficult to generate solid conclusions (Tellnes 1989a). A paper from many years ago reported that at least 41 different measurements of absence from work had been used in the past (Chadwick-Jones, Brown & Nicholson 1973). In the literature published on sickness certification in general practice at least 11 different measurements have been used (Tellnes 1989a). The epidemiology of sickness absence and social security is still a basic method used in this field of research (Brage & Ihlebæk 2009). Therefore, it has been recommended recently, by Hensing (2009), that only five different measurements should be used: frequency, length, cumulative incidence, incidence rate, and duration. These five measurements can be seen as a summary of measurements used in different studies and an application of epidemiologic methods in sickness absence research. There are opportunities to increase the quality of sickness absence research through an increased awareness of the importance of measurements. The same is true for concepts and definitions used in the field of sickness certification research (Tellnes 1989a). Though many new studies have been published during the last years, there is still a need for standardized reporting of sickness certification and sickness absence (Wynne-Jones et al. 2008).

The experience from the Buskerud study (Tellnes 1990) shows that the measurements used should reflect the area of practice or policy in which the findings of the studies are most likely to be used:

Incidence data of sickness certification may be used as an indicator for health problems (Tellnes & Bjerkedal 1989; Tellnes et al. 1989).

Duration data may be used for evaluation of rehabilitation (Tellnes 1989b).

Days lost data used for planning of prevention of health problems (Tellnes 1989c; Tellnes, Bruusgaard & Sandvik 1990).

To understand the nature of sickness certification, occupational rehabilitation, function, and work ability, it is also very important to use qualitative methods as well as philosophical methods in future research.

Brage et al. (1995) indicates that questions about illness, rather than about disease, could give higher estimates of the prevalence of disorders and health problems in population surveys. In the International Classification of Primary Care (ICPC), the 'reason for encounter' of a general practitioner, i.e. symptoms and illness experienced by patients, is classified by a number corresponding to each organic system (1–29). This classification should be useful for future population-based surveys in the field of sickness certification. Brage (1998) also reminds us that high work demands contribute to the large inter-occupational differences in sickness absence rates. He therefore recommends that employees with musculoskeletal health problems be given tasks that are adjusted and adapted to the individual's work capacity. Such adjustments of the workplace might reduce the need for future disability pensioning.

Assessment of function and work ability

Disease, illness, reduced function, and reduced functional ability are key concepts in sickness absence research (Reiso et al. 2001; Reiso et al. 2003). There is a growing interest in assessments of function and work ability because these assessments probably can supplement information about disease and illness, particularly in making decisions about sickness benefits, rehabilitation actions and disability pension, or in predicting duration of sickness absence.

Reiso's (2004) study supports the findings of Brage (1998), namely, that it is worth listening to the patient's self-assessment in the field of sickness absence. The patients' self assessed work ability was the most accurate predictor after three months of sickness absence. Depending upon the nature of the health problem, patients with high probability of intermediate and long-term sickness absence should be offered increased follow-up efforts by doctors and social insurance officers. On the other side, Reiso recommends that persons with high probability of short-term sickness absence should not be offered extensive rehabilitation measures.

A new methodology for work ability assessments was implemented by The National Labour and Welfare Administration (NAV) in Norway during the winter of 2010. The purpose was to provide an early assessment of work possibilities, resources, and barriers by involving the persons certified sick. In this context, the structured functional assessment method described by Østerås (2009) may provide a feasible way of transferring relevant information from the general practitioner to the NAV-employed executive officers, who make decisions with regards to workplace adjustments, rehabilitation, and social security benefits.

Since the middle of the 1990's, there has been a paradigmatic debate within Norwegian social insurance medicine concerning the biomedical concept of disease and the social function of social insurance medicine (Solli 2007). Among other results, Solli concluded his study as follows:

> A complex *functional ability model* is proposed which modifies and completes the biomedical model used in the WHO's International Classification of Functioning, Disability, and Health (ICF), by incorporating a proposed *complex medical model for health and disease*. *Significant activity limitation* is proposed as a new refinement of the criterion *injury to person*. It should replace *disease, injury, or defect*. The complex functional ability model is considered consistent both with the criterion *real equality of opportunity for everybody* and *the medical holistic criterion of objectivity*.

Nordenfelt (2008) has recently published a systematic analysis of the concept of work ability. The analysis is particularly focused on the following three contexts: medical insurance, training for a vocation or a profession, and evaluation of a job seeker. The ICF (WHO 2001) is described and discussed in the first chapter of Lorenfelt's book. The second chapter includes a description of the Norwegian function assessment scale (NFAS). In Norway, both ICF and NFAS are mostly used for research (Østerås 2009). However, there is still a need for developing tools or instruments for function and work ability assessments to be used by doctors, especially general practitioners.

Solli and da Silva (2010) analysed the holistic claims of the biopsychosocial conception of WHO's ICF. They propose a pluralistic-holistic ontology to make the complexity of ICF more coherent, action-oriented, and practically relevant.

Learning as a method in the return to work process

Illness and disease are the starting points for sickness absence, and the focus has traditionally been more on diagnosis and treatment of health problems than on factors that enhance the process of returning to work. Haugli and Steen (2001) evaluated a group learning program using a phenomenological understanding of body and disease and a mindfulness-based cognitive approach. The educational method was inspired by personal construct theory, which calls attention to human beings' capacity to redefine and reconstruct the meanings of any situation and symptom. This context emphasized an understanding of the body as a talking subject rather than focusing on pain and diagnosis; it considered the wholeness of participants' situations rather than viewing chronic muscular pain as either physical or psychological; it focused on each participant's and the whole group's resources, potentials and possibilities; and it challenged the participants to evoke their inner authority and internal validation. The findings underscore the relevance of considering psychological distress in chronic pain patients, not least as an important factor in helping pain patients to remain in the work force. These results show the relevance of developing experience and process-oriented group learning programs, in which the meditation method of 'mindfulness' and a focus on resources and potentials are emphasised. In order to facilitate this process, the training of health personnel in mindfulness-based cognitive approaches seems necessary.

From inactivity to action

Studies show that most occupational rehabilitation interventions should be carried out at the local level and in close contact with the workplace and primary health care personnel (Franche et al. 2005). However, people with more complex health conditions need more comprehensive occupational rehabilitation. The complexity of such interventions may improve function and work ability along many outcome dimensions, including physical endurance and strength, flexibility, body awareness, increased self-understanding, and coping skills, as well as understanding of the pain process. Occupational rehabilitation interventions should be directed both towards helping patients on long-term sickness absence to improve their level of functioning so as to regain and improve their work ability and towards changing the direction of their focus from symptoms and disability to an increased awareness of self, their own inherent resources, potentials, and competences. Medical knowledge alone does not seem to be sufficient to help get people back to work. Health personnel also need competence in educational methods with an emphasis on resource-oriented communication to counsel patients to increase their self-understanding.

The opinion of The National Labour and Welfare Administration (NAV), however, is that the workplace is the most suitable arena for follow-up of sickness absence, with the employer and the employees as the most important participants (Damberg 2009). In 2010, the 'work ability assessment benefit' (AAP) was introduced as a modification to the previous three benefits: rehabilitation benefit, vocational training benefit, and time-limited disability benefit. The AAP is based on a new working method internal to NAV. In this new setting, the doctors' work ability assessment is not as central as it used to be, and the general practitioners are now mostly asked by NAV to document the patients' health status or diagnoses. If this practice is implemented by NAV in the future, the consequence may be a reversal of the process of getting a more holistic assessment from doctors' sickness certification practices.

The recently introduced practice in NAV is not in accordance with a governmental group of experts that gave their report on sickness absence in February 2010 to the Ministry of Labour in Norway (Mykletun 2010). In this report, the proposal was to make it a duty for the doctors to assess patients work ability and degree of incapacity for work.

The challenge with this new policy from NAV is that the activities which enable a return to work need to take place in an extended arena, and not only in workplaces. Recent research indicates that multidisciplinary occupational rehabilitation programs significantly improved perceived work ability when compared with treatment as usual (Braathen, Veierstad & Heggenes 2007). Beyond this, persons with chronic health problems need inspiration and motivation to get healthier and return to work. Such aspects are described in more detail in chapter 12, which refers to evaluation studies that supports health-promoting nature and culture activities as a method of rehabilitation for persons to improve their quality of life and function (Batt-Rawden & Tellnes 2005; Tellnes 2009).

The findings above underline the importance of looking, not only at illness and disease from a pathological perspective, but at salutogenic activities that can positively promote peoples' health and capacity for work as well. Such methods seem to be the future in the field of social medicine and welfare in order to get people out of their roles of being certified sick and to increase their work ability and wellbeing.

Unfortunately, the dominant research on sickness absence has focused on how we should reduce health problems and make work-related arrangements to persons certified sick back to work. These approaches do not address the question of why people become certified sick in the first place. It seems reasonable to conclude that if we focus on this question in the light of a nature-culture-health perspective (NaCuHeal) (Tellnes 2009), we are in a better position to understand not only some of the most fundamental causes of long-term sickness absence, but also why so many people are able to live a normal and reasonably healthy life. Most importantly, this approach promises to give us a better understanding of why people are able to work and why they find their work meaningful.

References

Alexanderson, K. 2005. 'Research on sickness absence and disability pension'. Tellnes G, ed.: *Urbanization and health – new challenges in health promotion and prevention.* Oslo, Unipub (Oslo Academic Press), 306–315

Batt-Rawden, K.B. & Tellnes, G. 2005. 'Nature-culture-health activities as a method of rehabilitation: an evaluation of participant's health, quality of life and function'. *Int J Rehabiltation Research*, 28, 175–180

Braathen, T.N., Veierstad, K.B. & Heggenes, J. 2007. 'Improved work ability and return to work following vocational multidisciplinary rehabilitation of subjects on long-term sick leave'. *J Rehabil Med* 39, 493–499

Brage, S., Haldorsen E.M.H. et al. 1995. 'Assessment of sickness certification and concepts of musculoskeletal disease and illness in the general population'. *Scand J Prim Health Care*; 13, 1988–96

Brage, S. 1998. *Musculoskeletal health problems and sickness absence – an epidemiological study of concepts, determinants and consequences* (Thesis). Oslo, Institute of General Practice and Community Medicine, University of Oslo

Brage S. &, Ihlebæk, C. eds. 2009. 'Tema: Trygdeepidemiologi' (The Epidemiology of Social Insurance). *Nor J Epidemiol* 19, 101–234.

Chadwick-Jones, J.K., Brown, C.A. & Nicholson, N. 1973. 'Absence from work'. *Int Rev Appl Psychol*, 22, 137–154

Damberg, G. 2009. '«From inactivity to action» – a review of development and changes in the national insurance scheme in recent years'. *Nor J Epidemiol* 19,139–46

Franche, R.L., Baril, R. et al. 2005. 'Workplace-based return-to-work interventions: optimizing the role of stakeholders in implementation and research'. *J Occup Rehabil* 15, 525–542, available from: PM:16254753

Haugli, L. & Steen, E. 2001. *Kroniske muskel/skjelettsmerter og selvforståelse. Utvikling og evaluering av læringsmodell som vektlegger kroppen som meningsbærer.* (Chronic musculoskeletal pain and self-understanding. Development and evaluation of a teaching model emphasing mindfulness and embodiment) (Thesis). Oslo, Universitet i Oslo. In Norwgian

Hensing, G. 2009. 'The measurements of sickness absence – a theoretical perspective'. *Nor J Epidemiol* 19, 147–151

Mykletun, A. et al. 2010. *Tiltak for reduksjon i sykefravær: Aktiviserings- og nærværsreform. Ekspertgrupperapport til Arbeidsdepartementet 01.02.10 ifølge mandat av 27.11.09.* (How to reduce sickness absence). In Norwegian

Nordenfelt, L. 2008. *The concept of work ability.* Brussels, P.I.E. Peter Lang.

Reiso, H., Nygård, J.F. et al. 2001. 'Work ability and duration of certified sickness absence'. *Scand J Public Health*; 29, 218–225

Reiso, H., Nygård, J.F., et al. 2003. 'To ask the right question at the right time: When is the patient's self-assessed work ability most accurate as a predictor of the remaining duration of certified sickness absence?' *Nor J Epidemiology*; 13, 297–302

Reiso, H. 2004. *Work ability and sickness absence – A follow-up study in general practice* (Thesis). Oslo, Department of General Practice and Community Medicine, University of Oslo

Solli, H.M. 2007. *Justice, objectivity and disability assessment within social insurance medicine. An ethical and scientific-philosophical analysis of three disability models, seen in a historical perspective* (Thesis). Michael 4,193–520. www.dnms.no/index.php?seks_id=117216&treeRoot=117202&element=Subsek3&a=1

Solli, H.M. & Barbosa da Silva, A. 2010. 'The holistic claims of the biopsychosocial conception of WHO's International Classification of Functioning, Disability, and Health (ICF). A conceptual analysis on the basis of a pluralistic-holistic view of the human being'. *J Med Philos.* In press

Tellnes, G. 1989a. 'Sickness certification in general practice: a review'. *Family Practice* 6, 58–65

Tellnes, G. & Bjerkedal, T. 1989. 'Epidemiology of sickness certification'. *Scand J Soc Med* 17, 245–51

Tellnes, G., Svendsen, K-O. B. et al. 1989. 'Incidence of sickness certification'. *Scand J Prim Health Care* 7, 111–7

Tellnes, G. 1989b. 'Duration of episodes of sickness certification'. *Scand J Prim Health Care* 7, 237–44

Tellnes, G. 1989c. 'Days lost by sickness certification'. *Scand J Prim Health Care* 7, 245–51

Tellnes, G., Bruusgaard, D., & Sandvik, L. 1990. 'Occupational factors in sickness certification'. *Scand J Prim Health Care* 8, 37–44

Tellnes, G., Sandvik, L. & Moum, T. 1990. 'Inter-doctor variation in sickness certification'. *Scand J Prim Health Care* 8, 45–52

Tellnes, G. 1990. *Sickness certification – an epidemiological study related to community medicine and general practice* (Thesis). Oslo, University of Oslo, Department of Community Medicine

Tellnes, G. 2009. 'How can nature and culture promote health?' *Scand J Public Health* 37, 559–561. Editorial

WHO 2001. *International Classification of Functioning, Disability and Health: ICF*. Geneva, World Health Organization

Wynne-Jones, G., Mallen, C.D. et al. 2008. 'Rates of sickness certification in European primary care: A systematic review'. *Eur J Gen Pract* 14, 99–108

Østerås, N. 2009. *Functional assessments – A study on functional ability in a population, and structured assessments in general practice* (Thesis). Oslo, Institute of General Practice and Community Medicine, University of Oslo

Chapter 6

Disease, illness and long term sickness absence: A conceptual framework for categorising controversial cases

Halvor Nordby

Summary

The triad *disease*, *illness* and *sickness* can be used to clarify grey cases of long-term sickness absence – cases in which it is not obvious whether an absentee should be, or has to be, absent from work. The social concept of *sickness* applies in all the controversial cases, but this social dimension can be understood in different ways. Many cases of sickness absence involve states of negative first-person experience (illness) but no traditional somatic or mental disorder. However, there are other important categories as well, such as disease without subjective feeling of illness and sickness without illness or disease. The chapter argues that a critical analysis of long-term sickness absence on the basis of the concepts disease, illness and sickness has two normative implications. First, it constitutes a conceptual framework for categorisation and theoretical research on long-term sickness absence. Second, the analysis is useful politically and practically as a basis for developing system-related guidelines and 'conceptual tools' for securing communication with absentees.

Introduction

Recently, there has been a lot of political, public, and academic focus on long-term sickness absence. The reason is easy to understand. In many countries, there has been, within the last decades, a significant increase in the official number of people who are not working due to health problems. In many of the 'new' cases, absentees experience ill-health that cannot be traced to traditional somatic diseases. Understanding absentees' 'lifeworlds', their experienced illnesses, and modern 'lifestyle' diseases are not merely medical challenges. Why are so many people absent from work due to psycho-social problems and states, like burnout, chronic fatigue syndrome, and depression? What can be done to prevent and reduce long-term sickness absence caused by mental illness and social aspects of health problems? To what extent can work absence be explained by reference to absentees' personal values, attitudes, and social relations? These questions have psychological, sociological, and economical dimensions that go beyond the boundaries of traditional medicine (see chapters 3 and 4 above).

Many of the critical questions surrounding long-term sickness absence correspond to a well-known philosophical debate about the nature of disease. This debate has often focused on 'grey' cases of disease, states like fibromylgia, whip lash, ME, mild mental illness, and long-lasting undiagnosed pains (Nordenfelt 2001; Nordby 2006; chapter 2). As Worhall & Worhall (2001, 33) observe, these states are 'conditions whose status as diseases or not is controversial or intuitively unclear ahead of systematic analysis'. The hope has been that if we can use conceptual analysis to develop a general definition of the concept *disease*, then we can use that definition to determine how the difficult grey cases should be judged (Nordby 2006).

The same strategy can be used in a critical analysis of long-term sickness absence. Such an analysis will seek to shed light on controversial cases by clarifying whether they involve an *entitlement* to sickness absence. As an initial example, consider an otherwise healthy person who is absent from work due to work-related social problems. These problems, we may imagine, cause a negative subjective experience of illness in a wide sense. Furthermore, the person is socially sick in the formal sense that he has a medical sickness certificate; this label gives him social rights and exempts him from certain duties (Parsons

1951). But none of this is equivalent to having a traditional somatic or psychological disorder. It is therefore not *a priori* evident that a 'medical sickness certificate' *should* be granted to the absentee. In Norway, all doctors must consider sickness in relation to reduced work ability and the patient's job situation. It is not sufficient merely to confirm a health problem. Even so, the expression, 'medical sickness certificate', does indicate, after all, a *medical* judgment.

The aim in this chapter is to argue that the triad of disease, illness and sickness can help us to understand this and other grey cases of long-term sickness absence. According to an influential understanding, the triad corresponds to three perspectives on human ailment. As observed by Hoffmann in chapter 2 (above),

> ... disease is negative bodily occurrences as conceived of by the medical profession. Illness is negative bodily occurrences as conceived of by the person himself. Correspondingly, sickness is negative bodily occurrences as conceived of by the society and/or its institutions.

This traditional understanding, I will argue, provides a sound philosophical starting point for a critical analysis of long-term sickness absence.[1] However, we need a more fine-grained conception in order to fully understand the controversial cases. We need, in particular, to distinguish between different concepts of disease and different concepts of illness. For instance, disease is typically, but not necessarily, accompanied by a negative first-person experience, like dizziness, nausea, or pain (Nordby 2004). Furthermore, it is not obvious that disease without illness always warrants sickness absence: A person can be diagnosed with a disease that has not (so far) caused relevant functional disability or a reduced sense of well-being.

I will argue that a critical analysis of long-term sickness absence has normative consequences on two levels. First, the analysis constitutes a conceptual framework for understanding and discussing social phenomana related to disease and ill-health. Such a framework can be useful in empirical investigations and theoretical discussions of social mechanisms related to long-term sickness absence. Second, the analysis can be useful for political, practical,

---

[1] In chapter 2, Hofmann outlines a more detailed analysis of the concepts *disease*, *illness* and *sickness*. If not already acquainted with these concepts, the reader should read his discussion before embarking on this chapter.

and communicative purposes. It can be used to develop norms on a system level and to understand how health professionals and social workers should secure communication with absentees on an individual level.

Background

Sometimes it is not obvious whether an absentee has to be, or should be, away from work. In such cases, the absentee does not have a traditional somatic or psychological disease that has a significant impact on his subjective well-being or functional abilities related to his work. The cause of the person's absence is instead more complex and can typically be traced to demanding psycho-social working conditions and first-person negative experiences of illness (Michie & Williams 2003; see also chapter 3 above). But then the question arises: Is it really necessary for the absentee to be away from work? Or, formulated more explicitly in a normative way, is such a person *entitled* to be absent?

Empirical studies of long-term sickness absence have been pursued in different ways. Extensive research has offered comprehensive insights into categories of absentees and processes leading to long-term sickness absence. However, qualitative and quantitative empirical approaches are not the only possible strategies for understanding why so many people are absent from work for longer periods. An alternative strategy is to analyse long-term sickness absence more critically. Such a strategy will seek to understand the concept *long-term sickness absence* philosophically, in the light of general theories of human ailment and psycho-social processes. The aim is to help us to understand not only how the concept actually is applied, but how it *should* be applied.

The present discussion pursues this overall strategy. It aims to understand controversial cases by thinking of them as grey cases. Here I use terminology that is often used in discussions of the nature of disease. The idea is as follows: The concept *disease* clearly applies to a number of negative bodily states. AIDS, cancer, myocardial infarction, arthritis, measles, tuberculosis and diabetes are uncontroversial paradigm cases of disease. It is equally clear that the concept disease does not apply to many bodily states a person can be in, even to states that can affect well-being or normal functioning. Qualitative states like a headache, tiredness, or stiffness are often not regarded as disease or symptoms of disease. The same applies to many physical states that are not always accompanied by conscious discomfort to any significant extent. A scratch or a minor injury is not a 'disease' in an intuitive sense of the word.

In addition to the clear 'black' and 'white' cases, there are cases of widespread uncertainty or disagreement. Mild mental illnesses like 'burn-out' are often considered to be grey cases. Other controversial cases include fibromyalgia, whip lash, lower back pain, and chronic fatigue syndrome. Grey cases often arise from a long-lasting negative subjective experience, like pain, in which the medical profession has been unable to identify an underlying physical and/or pathological cause.

The fundamental motivation for analysing disease has been the need for arriving at reasonable verdicts about the grey cases (Worhall & Worhall 2001; Nordby 2006). Consider a doctor who tells an absentee that it has not been possible to locate an underlying physical cause for the pain he has experienced in his lower back for a long time. The absentee asks if this means that he does not have a disease. For him, it is important to know whether the label 'disease' applies to him. The doctor, however, finds it difficult to give the absentee a clear yes-or-no answer. The (quite ambitious) hope has been that a careful conceptual analysis of the concept of disease can clarify its conceptual content, so that it becomes clearer to the medical profession how this and other grey cases should be judged:

> Perhaps philosophers, with their expertise in conceptual matters, can provide significant help here by providing a clear-cut and defensible characterisation, not of any particular disease (that seems clearly a scientific issue), but of the class of diseases – of what might be called 'disease-in-general' (Worhall & Worhall 2001, 33).

The idea has been that a general characterisation of the concept of disease can make it easier to understand how the disputed grey states should be categorised. If it turns out that the concept applies to a given bodily state, then it is a 'black' positive case of disease. If the state does not meet the condition of the definition, then it is a 'white' negative case, i.e. not a disease.

I have so far focused on disease, but the idea that conceptual analyses can shed light on basic health concepts is more comprehensive. All controversial health concepts can be addressed critically by using conceptual analysis (Nordby 2006). Other concepts that have been explored philosophically involve common concepts like *health*, *illness* and *sickness*, and more theoretical concepts like *quality of life, well-being* and *sense of coherence* (see chapter 12). In discussions of absenteeism, especially in the recent years, these concepts have in turn been linked to concepts like *motivation, working ability,* and *psycho-social working environment* (Nordenfelt 2008).

My focus here will be the concept of *long-term sickness absence*, but the task of exploring this concept is part of the overall strategy I have outlined. The aim is to use conceptual analysis to 'sharpen the boundaries of the concept' (Harman 1999), just as philosophers have attempted to analyse *disease*.

There is, at the same time, two crucial differences between the traditional analyses of *disease* and a critical analysis long-term sickness absence. First, the aim of the analyses of *disease* has been to clarify the nature of the ontological 'real-world' category of disease (Worhall & Worhall 2001, chapter 7). The aim of a critical analysis of the concept *long-term sickness absence*, on the other hand, should not be to determine what long-term sickness absence is. Determining when this concept applies is a straigthforward matter. It applies when a person is away from work for a sufficiently long time because she has a medical sickness certificate.[2] Just as the normative aim of the analyses of disease has been to determine when we should apply the term 'disease', the normative aim of the analysis of long-term sickness absence should be to determine when a person is entitled to long-term sickness absence. Thus, the (complex) object concept of the critical analysis is *entitlement* to long-term sickness absence.

Entitlement is here understood as a kind of epistemic warrant which is a broader notion than justification. Corresponding to widespread philosophical opinion, I will assume that an entitlement does not require a consciously held justification. Entitlement is a more comprehensive concept than justification. The traditional idea has been that

> ... the notion of epistemic warrant is broader than the ordinary notion of justification. An individual's epistemic warrant may consist in a justification that the individual has for a belief or other epistemic act or state. But it may also be an *entitlement* that consists in a status of operating in an appropriate way in accord with

---

[2] There are some different views about the differences between short-term and long-term sickness absence. The crucial question is how many days an absentee must be away from work for the latter concept to apply. The point is that once this is formally decided in a given country or region, it is unproblematic to determine whether a case of sickness absence constitutes long-term sickness absence.

norms of reasons, even when these norms cannot be articulated by the individual who has the status (Burge 1996, 93, original italics).

Thus, a person might be entitled to be absent from work without being able to state all the underlying reasons that actually justify the absence. An absentee will, for instance, typically not have detailed knowledge of all relevant medical aspects of the disease or injury that justify the absence.

The second key difference between an analysis of disease and an analysis of long-term sickness absence is that the latter should not aim to analyse conceptual meaning. The reason is obvious: It is not difficult to understand what the expression 'long-term sickness absence' *means* in our public language. The concept that the expression denotes has a conceptual content (intension) with reasonably clear boundaries (extension). As argued above, what is not so clear is what it takes to have an entitlement to long-term sickness absence. This is a normative question about valid reasons. Thus, insofar as the aim of the conceptual analysis is to analyse conceptual meaning, it is the word 'entitlement' that is the crucial expression (Peacocke 1996). The aim is to analyse the meaning of 'entitlement' within this specific area.

Categories of disease, illness and sickness

When the concept long-term sickness absence applies, this often happens in the following way: A person has an experience of illness or other bodily symptoms that indicate an underlying health problem. He goes to his doctor who discovers a disease that justifies long-term sickness absence. The person becomes a patient and is given a sickness certificate issued by the doctor (see chapter 2).

Thus, the most straightforward example includes all the three concepts. Grey cases of long-term sickness absence, as I have characterised them, differ from the most straightforward example in the sense that it is not evident that all the three concepts apply in the typical way. Here the term 'typical' refers to different possibilities. There are many ways in which grey cases can differ from *paradigm cases*, in which it is evident that a person really is entitled to long-term sickness absence.

Notice that a paradigm case does not have to involve a documented traditional somatic or psychological disease. A person's entitlement to be absent from work for a longer period may be grounded in external relations to close relatives who have serious health problems. A typical example might be a parent who has a child with a serious disease or injury.

However, even when an absentee's entitlement is related to the individual, he does not need to have a documented traditional disease. If a person experiences long-lasting and severe pain, then this is clearly sufficient for legitimate work absence. So illness does not have to be combined with 'objective' disease in order to warrant long-term sickness absence. Serious, long-lasting, and negative experiences qualify for sickness even though a disease cannot be documented in an intersubjective way (Carel 2008). Strong *sensational* illnesses involving pain are clearly sufficient for long-term sickness absence.[3] It does not matter how this kind of illness is related to disease or injury.

Mild sensational illness is less straightforward. If I have a mild headache one day, perhaps due to a social gathering the previous night – and if this can be relieved with a common medicament like paracetamol – then it is far from evident that I am entitled to being absent from work. Long-term sickness absence is more problematic. If I have mild headache that lasts for several days or even weeks, it is not clear that I should go to work, even if the headache can be relieved with medicaments. A chronic headache is normally a sign that 'something is wrong', and that curative treatment, possibly in a wide interpersonal sense, is appropriate.

Furthermore, in order to relieve mild sensational illness, it is sometimes necessary to focus on demanding physical or psycho-social working conditions. Heavy workloads and experiences of not being able to 'fulfill all expectations' can cause stress and negative experiences like headaches and pains (see for instance chapters 8 and 11). So, depending on the situation, cases involving absentees who have mild sensational illness often constitute grey cases of long-term sickness absence. These cases are not as clear as those involving stronger illnesses.

I have so far focused on sensational illnesses involving pain – illnesses that include a negative first-person experience with a determinate qualitative content. This kind of illness should be distinguished from *existensial* illness

---

[3] There is a comprehensive philosophical literature on the nature of sensational conscious episodes, see e.g. Guttenplan (2000); Gertler & Shapiro (2007). For the purposes of this chapter, it is not necessary to focus on the philosophical discussions. It is sufficient to define a sensation as a subjective experience that has a determinate emotional content for the subject.

– illness that is difficult to 'pin down' to a single negative conscious episode with a determinate emotional content. Existential illness constitutes a significant part of a person's world view – his cognitive perspective on himself and the world around him. This alternative concept of illness refers to a lack of motivation, a loss of personal strength to do everyday tasks, and a feeling that one cannot cope with all the things one is expected to cope with (chapter 11). Existential illness can involve a genuine feeling that life has no meaning ('What is the purpose of it all?') or a fundamental feeling of emptiness or loneliness (Nagel 1979).

Variations on what I call 'existential illness' are described theoretically and empirically in many other chapters of this book. As the research shows, an absentee can experience this form of illness in different ways. However, what the experiences have in common is that they do not have a strong qualitative content like the experience of pain, nausea, or dizziness. The subjective element is much more vague and difficult to articulate, but it can nevertheless be the cause of reduced quality of life and diminished 'sense of coherence' (see chapter 12).

Can existential illness sometimes be a legitimate reason for long-term sickness absence? The answer is clearly yes. Personal grief can be a good reason for being absent from work for a longer period. Psychological crisis is another category. If one of my closest relatives experience sudden and acute loss of health, this will normally have a significant and dramatic psychological impact on my well-being and ability to perform everyday tasks (Nordby & Nøhr 2008).

However, other cases are clearly more problematic, and sometimes existensial illness seems insufficient for entitlement to long-term sickness absence. Consider a person who thinks that his 'daily work' has 'no real meaning'. Such a personal experience that 'boring' routine work makes it impossible to realise one's personal potential is not sufficient for entitlement to sickness absence. So too with conflicting interests, value tensions, and fundamental desires to live one's life in alternative ways. The desire to have a year off in order to 'do something else', like travelling around the world, cannot be a valid reason for having a medical sickness certificate.

In patient communication, it is often important for doctors to make a clear distinction between somatic disease and illness experiences, especially when a medical sickness certificate is given on the basis of illness that leads to reduced relevant work ability (Reiso 2004; Østerås 2009; Kamaleri et al. 2009). The reason is that a medical sickness certificate can strengthen an absentee's belief that she is a person with a 'genuine disease' – it can contribute to a 'medicalization' of personal problems that are not health problems in a traditional somatic sense.

Consider for instance a person who goes to his doctor because he is feeling depressed. He is given a medical sickness certificate, and he thinks to himself, 'Now it has been confirmed what I have known all the time (and what the others doubted), that I am a person with a health problem who really needs proper medical treatment'. Consequently, the person becomes a patient (at least from his own perspective), and he feels, in fact, worse than what he did when he went to the doctor in the first place.

However, the doctor has done nothing more than to assess the patient's illness and work ability as a way to determine sickness (Reiso 2004). The patient's cognitive perspective is changed, but the underlying condition remains the same (Carel 2008). In other words, the label 'medical sickness certificate' does not give the patient a justification for thinking that the physical nature of his own body state has changed. This is an importnant point, since it is possible for doctors to ground medical sickness certificates in experiences of illness that are not accompanied by traditional somatic or psyhological disorder.[4] Indeed, this is precicely what happens nowadays in many of the controversial grey cases of long-term sickness absence.

Disease

In a critical discussion of long-term sickness absence, illness without a documented traditional disease is the most important category. But grey cases of long-term sickness absence can also arise in other ways.

Sometimes a disease is discovered without any subjective symptoms of illness. It is not uncommon that screening, routine tests, or somatic symptoms uncover an underlying disease. A typical case might be breast cancer that is disovered in mammography. Similarly, a patient who has a mild long-lasting cough but no real illness might be diagnosed with lung cancer after a MRI of his chest.

---

[4] In Norway, the form that is used in classification in primary care can be found at www.kith.no.

In both of these examples, it is reasonable to assume that the person is entitled to long-term sickness absence if he so desires. The reason is that cancer is a very serious disease - it has often fatal consequences in the sense that the patient is at risk of dying quite soon. Although the physiological effect are (for the moment) undramatic and have no direct sensational consequences for the patient, the psychological implictions are so dramatic that he is entitled to be absent from work, at least for some time. In short, to get the message that tests have revealed a very serious disease will often lead to a personal existensial crisis that clearly warrants long-term sickness absence, if this is in the patient's best interests. Very serious disease clearly belongs within the black positive cases that justify long-term sickness absence.

Many diseases are not as as serious as cancer, but they can nevertheless have dramatic negative consequences for individual patients. Examples include hypertension, extreme obesity, multiple sclerosis, arthiritis, and many musculoskeletal problems that are difficult to control and cure with traditional medical treatment. If these diseases are treated correctly, the prospects for recovery, or a reasonably good level of functional abilities and well-being for many years, are often good. Furthermore, many diseases, if treated properly, are not very serious, not even in the long run. I think we have equally clear intuitions about these diseases, but now in the white negative direction. Imagine a person who has a disease which does not have serious consequences if controlled in the right way, who does not experience illness, and whose disease does not affect relevant working abilitites; such a person is not entitled to long-term sickness absence.

Here the concept of 'working ability' is important (Reiso 2004; Nordenfelt 2008; Østerås 2009). Getting absentees back to work can often be a matter of making practical arrangmens, and the ability to work will depend on the nature of the work in question. If a postman has a fractured leg, he is entitled to long-term sickness absence if he cannot do alternative work at his workplace. But if an acedemic lecturer has the same kind of injury, it is far from clear that he cannot perform his daily work. It is not necessary to be able to walk without crutches to give lectures or to write books and articles. The same point about work ability applies when a person has a disease. A person with a heart disease should not do his daily work if this work involves stress or physical strain. But he can often do alternative work that is less demanding physically or mentally.

Notice that these inferences can only be valid when a person has a disease that does not involve illness. If the disease has begun to cause negative subjective experience, loss of well-being, and reduced working ability, the picture becomes more complicated. But our focus now is on disease without illness - neither sensational nor existential - and within this restricted focus the above analyses seem sound.

Other categories

What about sickness without disease or illness? In the most fundamental sense of sickness – when sickness is understood as equivalent to having a medical sick certificate – this is a genuine logical possibility. The obvious reason is that it is, in principle, possible for a person without illness to pretend that he experiences illness. From an 'outsider perspective', others cannot directly observe a person's inner mental states (see chapter 12). The third-person – first-person distinction implies that a person without illness can be given the label 'sick' even though he does not really experience a health problem. Consequently, sickness fraud is mentioned by Hofmann as a possibility in chapter 2 above.

Must sickness without personal experience of illness or disease always involve fraud? Obviously not, as long as sickness absence can be grounded in *external* relations to close relatives who experience ill-health. But if we restrict our focus and consider cases in which the source of sickness is the *individual*, the category becomes more murky and suspicious. Remember that we have made a distinction between different forms of illness, between mild and strong, and between sensational and existential illness. Sickness together with existential illness – illness in the most holistic sense - is therefore a genuine possibility.

Within the category of sickness without disease or illness, sickness cannot be accompanied by *any* kind of illness. And then it seems reasonable to assume that the person with the medical sickness certificate is not really entitled to long-term sickness absense. If a person does not experience any health problems that can be related to disease or illness, then his or her own mental and physical states – considered in isolation from the psycho-social environment – do not constitute a sound basis for work absence due to health problems.

There is another form of sickness that should be mentioned. A person who thinks he should be absent from work might be working because he has not been given a medical sickness certificate. He might nevertheless be acknowledged as a person who should not work from the perspective of his family, friends, or collegues. In these cases, the formal concept of sickness does not apply from the social institution that the medical profession represents. The person nevertheless falls under the general idea of sickness in the wider sense that he is, from an alternative social perspective, acknowledged as a person with sickness (Gannik & Launsø 2000). There is, in short, an incompatibility between different social perspectives on the person's state of health (Helman 2007).

An interesting question in these cases is whether the application of sickness from the alternative perspective can be sufficient for applying disease or illness. This does not seem to be a genuine possibility. A person's status as a person with sickness cannot *be* an illness or a disease – other persons' *thoughts* about a person cannot be *identical* to a negative bodily state with a real ontological or phenomenological nature that qualifies as a disease or an illness. To argue that cognitive acknowledgement by others is equivalent to disease or illness, and that this equivalence therefore warrants a medical sickness certificate, does not seem to be a valid argument.

I have so far focused on single occurrences of disease, illness and sickness. Combinations yield new possibilities. Consider the distinction between strong and mild sensational illness. I have argued that strong sensational illness clearly is a black positive case of entitlement to long-term sickness absence. Milder forms, however, are grey cases. So what about mild sensational illness together with disease? Does this give a stronger entitlement to long-term sickness absence?

The answer is not clear. Why should a person be more entitled to be away from work just because he knows that he has disease? It seems that mild illness has to be combined with disease that affects relevant work ability in order to constitute a stronger entitlement. So mild sensation illness combined with disease does not authomatically yield an entitlement to sickness absence.

Knowledge that one has a disease sometimes leads to existential worries. Knowledge of disease may therefore cause existensial illness. I argued above that existensial illness without disease is insufficient for entitlement to long-term sickness absence. When existensial illness is combined with disease, the situation becomes more complex. Existential worries related to acute loss of health belong in this category. This kind of illness – caused by an experienced psychological crisis – is strikingly different from existential illness caused by 'boring' routine work or an uninspiring life situation. But we still need to make a distinction between different forms of disease. Existential illness caused by a very serious disease like cancer clearly warrants long-term sickness absence, but a disease that is not serious does not seem to yield the same entitlement. Being worried about the future due to a diagnosis of arthiritis or coronary heart disease is not sufficient for entitlement to long-term sickness absence.

Generalisations

More could be said about combinations of disease, illness and sickness. This, however, falls outside the aims and limits here. The aim has been to show that if we use the triad disease, illness and sickness, then we have a good starting point for discussing controversial cases of long-term sickness absence. In short, the three concepts give us a useful vocabulary for talking about the difficult cases. But this require that we redefined the original concepts. If we use the concepts without dividing them into subclasses like sensational and existensial illness, it is impossible to capture and classify the grey cases of long-term sickness absence in a sufficiently refined way.

In addition to this general conceptual implication, I have developed normative conclusions about some of the most important categories. The main conclusions can be summed up in the following table, where 'black positive cases' means 'entitlement to long-term sickness absence'.

Categories/ classification	Black positive cases	Grey cases	White negative cases
Single occurrences	• Strong sensational illness • Disease that clearly affects relevant work ability	• Mild sensational illness • Disease with unclear implications for work ability	• Existential illness • Sickness • Disease that does not affect work ability
Combinations	• Existensial illness caused by serious disease • Mild sensational illness caused by serious disease		• Existential illness caused by disease that is (i) not serious and (ii) does not lead to reduced work ability

In the black cases, an absentee is normally entitled to long-term sickness absence if this is in his best interests. In other words, he can legitimately claim that his health problems undermine his ability to work, even when impaired work ability cannot be measured in a straightforward way. Similarly, in the white negative cases, the absentee's state of health is normally not a valid reason for being absent. The grey cases continue to be grey. Further analyses and probably even finer distinctions are needed to determine which side they fall on.

This classification can be used to formulate two important conditions on sickness absence. First, it defines conditions that are sufficient for being in the black, grey, and white categories. For instance, if a person has strong sensational illness, then this is sufficient for entitlement to long-term sickness absence (it does not matter how the other concepts apply). Second, the classification says something about necessary conditions. For instance, sickness alone cannot constitute a sound basis for long-term sickness absence. It is necessary that sickness is combined with one or both of the other concepts.

It should be emphasised that the main aim here has not been to develop final categories. The aim has been to show that by applying and refining the concepts disease, illness and sickness, both theorists and practitioners are in a better position to understand and talk about grey cases of long-term sickness absence. This should be accepted even by those who disagree with the tentative categories I have outlined.

There is, unfortunately, complete conceptual confusion in the literature on long-term sickness absence. In a very interesting review, Wikman et al. (2005, 453–4) explored a comprehensive number of publications and concluded that:

> ... in the debate about health, ill health, sickness, and sickness absence there is often a confusing use of different concepts. These different concepts are often used as interchangeable alternatives, although they are based on very different conceptual and material prerequisites ... In conclusion, the fact that illness, disease and sickness absence have been found to be so different in terms of magnitude and development over time shows the need for a very careful use of different concepts and indicators.

In the light of the fact that theorists have understood the basic concepts in strikingly different way, it is not surprising that there is so much disagreement about the controversial grey cases of long-term sickness absence. It is unfortunate if theorists in fact talk past each other when they think they really agree or disagree. In science, there should be agreement about the facts, but there should also be sufficient agreement about the meaning of the language that is used to talk about the facts. In this area, terminological issues seem to represent a significant obstacle to real progress.

The same point applies in health care communication involving absentees. In analyses of basic health concepts, the traditional aim has been to develop definitions that capture a common understanding – concepts with a meaning that both doctors and patients will defer to (Nordby 2008). So too with long-term sickness absence. A narrow stipulative concept with an idiosyncratic meaning that does not capture a common understanding that many people share will not be a concept with a wide, useful application in doctor-patient interaction and other communicative relations (Nordby 2006).

Consider as an example a patient who feels a little frustrated when his doctor says 'We have not been able to connect your symptoms to an underlying disease'. Hearing this statement, the patient forms the association that the doctor thinks he is not 'really ill', and he thinks to himself: 'Of course I have a disease. The fact that I am feeling ill and have all these other problems and symptoms *must* mean that I have a disease'. But the doctor, we can imagine, did not mean to question the patient's experiences. She meant to talk about somatic issues and thought the patient would be glad to hear that no pathological findings were made. It is reasonable to assume that if the patient had realised that the doctor intended to talk about this, then he would not have formed the negative beliefs about the doctor's statement.

I do not mean to argue that this is a very representative case, but it illustrates an important point: The framework outlined above can provide a more neutral ground for talking about controversial health problems and cases of sickness absence. We must not forget that good communication with absentees is a fundamental aim in many health and social care discourses that aim to understand and possibly reduce long-term sickness absence. If this communication is poor, then empirical knowledge – no matter how valid it is – is of limited value in real-life practices.

Conclusion

It is possible to critically analyse long-term sickness absence in the way theorists have analysed basic health concepts like *disease*. The crucial object concept of the analysis is the normative concept *entitlement* to long-term sickness absence. I have argued that the traditional triad of *disease*, *illness* and *sickness* constitute a promising starting point for exploring this concept. However, the triad needs to be refined in order to capture the disputed cases in an illuminating way. We need to distinguish various forms of disease, illness and sickness in order to develop a suitable conceptual framework for addressing the crucial normative questions.

This framework can be fruitful as a shared conceptual platform in public discussions, for academics and for health- and social workers who are engaged in communication with absentees. The framework makes it easier to develop important categories on a general level, and it can be used as a set of conceptual tools in one-to-one communication with absentees.

References

Burge, T. 1996. 'Our entitlement to self-knowledge'. *Proceedings of the Aristotelian society*, 91–116

Carel, H. 2008. *Illness*. Stocksfield, Acumen

Gannik, D. & Launsø, L. 2000. *Disease, knowledge and society*. Copenhagen, Samfundslitteratur

Gertler, B. & Shapiro, L. 2007. *Arguing about the mind*. London, Routledge

Guttenplan, S. 2000. *Mind's landscape*. Oxford, Blackwell

Helman, C. 2007. *Culture, health and illness*. London, Hodder Arnold

Kamaleri, Y. et al. 2009. 'Does the number of musculoskeletal pain sites predict work disability?' *European journal of pain*, 426–30

Michie, S. & Williams, S. 2003. 'Reducing work related psychological ill health and sickness absence: A systematic review'. *Occupational and environmental medicine*, 3–9

Nagel, T. 1979. *Mortal questions*. Cambridge, Cambridge University Press

Nordby, H. 2004. 'The importance of knowing how to talk about illness without applying the concept of illness'. *Nursing philosophy*, 30–40

Nordby, H. 2006. 'The analytic-synthetic distinction and conceptual analyses of basic health concepts'. *Medicine, health care and philosophy*, 169–80

Nordby, H. 2008. 'Medical explanations and lay conceptions of disease and illness in doctor-patient interaction'. *Theoretical medicine and bioethics*, 357–70

Nordby, H. & Nøhr, Ø. 2008. 'Communication and empathy in an emergency setting'. *Scandinavian journal of trauma, resuscitation and emergency medicine*, 1–6

Nordenfelt, L. 2001. *Health, science and ordinary language*. Amsterdam/New York NY, Rodopi

Nordenfelt, L. 2008. *The concept of work ability*. Brussels: P.I.E. Peter Lang

Parsons, T. 1951. 'Illness and the role of the physician: A sociological perspective'. *American journal of orthopsychiatry*, 452–60

Peacocke, C. 1996. 'Entitlement, self-knowledge and conceptual redeployment'. *Proceedings of the Aristotelian society*, 117–58

Reiso, H. 2004. *Work ability and sickness absence: A follow-up study in general practice*. D.Phil dissertation, The Faculty of Medicine, The University of Oslo

Wikman, A., Marklund, S. & Alexanderson, K. 2005. 'Illness, disease and sickness absence. An empirical test of differences between concepts of ill health'. *Journal of epidemial community health*, 450–54

Worrhall, J. & Worhall, J. 2001. 'Defining disease: Much ado about nothing?' Tymieniecka, A. & Agazzi, E. eds.: *Analecta Husserliana*, 33–55

Østerås, N. 2009. *Functional assessments: A Study of functional ability in a population, and structured assessments in general practice*. D.Phil dissertation. The Faculty of Medicine, The University of Oslo

Chapter 7

The subjectivity of illness, social roles and the harmful dysfunction analysis of disease

Halvor Nordby

Summary

Many controversial cases of long-term sickness absence involve genuine first-person negative experiences of illness that have not been traced to traditional disease states. But the fact that these cases do not involve documented disease in a traditional sense does not necessarily mean that they do not involve disease at all. This depends on how the general concept *disease* is defined. From an evaluative point of view, it is possible to accept that first-person negative experience is sufficient for disease. However, even theorists who have defended naturalistic definitions of disease can accept that the controversial cases involve disease. The chapter uses Wakefield's influential 'harmful dysfunction' definition of disease to show that it is possible for naturalists to accept that illness and a 'harmful' social role are sufficient for disease. I conclude that the question of whether illness and sickness can be sufficient for disease is a deep philosophical question one and outline some implications of this.

Introduction

Controversial cases of long-term sickness absence often involve absentees who experience forms of illness that are not accompanied by documented traditional diseases (chapters 2, 3 above). A typical example might be a person who is experiencing a mild form of undiagnosed pain in his back. Is the pain sufficiently regular and intense to warrant long-term sickness absence? If the pain is connected to working conditions, is it possible for the workplace to improve these conditions? In other cases, absentees have more indeterminate psychological experiences related to their overall subjective perspectives on themselves and on the world around them, experiences that cannot be reduced to direct and negative sensations of *qualia* (chapter 6). States in this category include chronic fatigue syndrome, social problems, existential experiences like grief, and many mild mental disorders.

Illness that has not been traced to a documented disease is not necessarily illness that is not caused by a disease (see chapter 2). Sometimes, further empirical investigations uncover undetected disease states. However, even when a patient's condition is sufficiently clarified, uncertainty may prevail. In these cases, the crucial question, far less tractable than empirical questions, is whether the health problem that is uncovered should be labelled a 'disease'. This is a metaphysical and philosophical question. It concerns the meaning of the word 'disease', how the general concept of disease should be defined and applied in controversial cases (Nordenfelt 2001; Nordby 2006).

Different perspectives on disease will address the controversial cases in different ways. There has been quite a lot of disagreement about the nature of disease, so this is not an area where we can turn to the literature or to 'experts' for uniform answers (Hofmann 2001; Lindstrøm 2009). However, there is one assumption that is commonly accepted in discussions of the nature of disease, illness and sickness. This assumption can be formulated as follows: Experienced illness and a sick role *cannot* be sufficient for disease.

According to this 'insufficiency assumption', as I will label it, there is a fundamental metaphysical difference between illness and disease. Illness, theorists have assumed, is essentially a phenomenological notion that refers to negative conscious episodes, loss of well-being, and reduced quality of life (Tellnes 1989; Fulford 1989; Nordby 2006). Disease, on the other hand, has commonly been thought to be a descriptive and objective state that can be observed in an intersubjective way (Hofmann 2001). The idea has been that it is possible to use our common language to formulate essential conditions for a state of ill-health to count as a disease (Nordenfelt 1993).

The aim of this chapter is to cast doubt on the insufficiency assumption. I will do this by discussing it in the light of evaluationism and naturalism, the two main traditions in the literature on the nature of disease. I will focus on central theories within these traditions and argue that these theories are consistent with the idea that illness and sickness can be sufficient for disease. This does not mean that the insufficiency assumption is false. But it shows that we are too hasty if we accept it on the basis of pretheoretical intuition, that there are good reasons for rejecting it, and that the questions about the nature of disease, illness and sickness are deep philosophical questions. In the final section I outline some practical consequences of these conclusions.

Disease, illness and sickness absence

Within recent philosophy of medicine and health care, it has been common to make a fundamental distinction between disease and illness. The idea has been that disease represents the medical profession's perspective on ill-health. Disease, understood like this, is a scientific, objective, and normative concept. Illness, on the other hand, has been thought of as subjective, private, and flexible. The standard assumption has been that the concept refers to experiences of being ill and the individual's first-person perspectives on ill-health (chapter 2; Tellnes 1989).

This distinction between disease and illness leaves open how disease and illness should be characterized metaphysically. All the distinction says is that we should make a distinction between two different perspectives on health problems. Exploring what is actually judged to be disease and illness from these two perspectives, on a specific or general level, requires a further step.

Many theorists have taken this further step when they have assumed that there is a more substantial metaphysical difference between disease and illness. Disease and illness have often been thought of as states with entirely different properties. Disease has been connected to what we might think of as *descriptivism* - the assumption that pathological disorders can be fully described in a public language. According to descriptivism, there is nothing more to the nature of disease than what can be captured in a proper definition of disease. Illness, on the other hand has been thought of as *phenomenological* concept that cannot be fully 'translated' into a common, shared language. The standard assumption has been that illness refers to the qualitative nature of negative first-person experiences – private experiences like pain, dizziness, and nausea (Nordby 2006, 2008).

Careal defines this phenomenological approach as 'health within illness' and describes it like this:

> Rather than measuring the experience of the ill person in objective parameters – how far from the norm she is – health within illness focuses on experiences of personal growth, adaption and rediscovery. A phenomenological approach enables the expression of these experiences in order to give a more complete description of the altered relationship of the ill person to her world and a better understanding of her experience (Careal 2008, 16).

The distinction between a 'reflective life world approach' and a physiological and 'objective' disease perspective has been conceived of as a deep philosophical distinction in many health care discourses and especially within the caring sciences (Dahlberg et al. 2001; Carrieri-Kohlman et al. 2003; Baillie 2005). Corresponding to widespread assumptions about the inexplicable and irreducible nature of human consciousness, it is often assumed that disease cannot fully explain the phenomenological nature of illness. Indeed, this is the reason why many have held that we should distinguish illness from disease. Even those who have sought to define disease have accepted that we need a concept of illness in addition to the descriptive concept of disease. They have not, after all, denied that patients can feel pain. The crucial question has rather been whether pain experiences and other states of illness can be fully understood and explained in a common language, in a way such that they meet a set of medical conditions and thereby 'deserve' the objective title *disease*. The standard view has been that this is impossible.

This general debate about the difference between illness and disease is relevant in discussions of many different health problems (Nordenfelt & Twaddle 1993). Especially interesting from a critical perspective are cases in which a person with an illness is attributed the social status of sickness in the sense that he has a medical sickness certificate. In these cases, both illness and sickness apply, but this does not happen in the typical way, that is, through the discovery of a disease which usually serves as a mediating concept (chapter 2). The epistemic link goes instead directly from illness to sickness.

This direct conceptual relationship can be explored from various perspectives, but it is not my aim here to compare these perspectives. For the present argumentative purposes, I will understand sickness as equivalent to having a sickness certificate. The important point is that this concept of sickness, like the scientific concept of disease, is a formal and objective concept (Tellnes 1989; Reiso 2004; Østerås 2009). Having a sickness certificate is a descriptive label with sharp boundaries. It is not difficult to understand when this concept has been applied to a person: It happens, in short, when the person has been given a sickness certificate.

Thus, in controversial cases of illness and sickness, there is a link between the private and the public – the personal and the descriptive. The crucial difference between the controversial cases and those involving documented traditional disease is that the former have not been 'legislated' by the medical profession. Doctors have not been able to identify an underlying 'objective' cause that warrants a sickness certificate. But does this mean that these controversial cases do not involve disease at all?

Strategies for clarifying basic health concepts

One way of exploring whether illness and sickness can be sufficient for disease is to analyze the concepts in the way philosophers have attempted to analyze other controversial concepts. Harman formulates the idea of conceptual analysis in an illuminating way:

> Typically, attempts at philosophical analysis proceed by the formulation of one or more tentative analyses ... [of the target concept]... and then the consideration of test cases. If exactly one of the proposed analyses does not conflict with 'intuitions' about any test cases, it is taken to be at least tentatively confirmed. Further research then uncovers new test cases in which intuitions conflict with the analysis. The analysis is then modified or replaced by a completely different one, which is in turn tested against imagined cases, and so on (Harman 1999, 139).

The traditional aim of a conceptual analysis is to locate and clarify a definition of a target concept that is 'hidden' in our common language, so that it becomes clearer how the concept applies (Nordenfelt 2001). If this can be done, then we can simply use the definition to understand how the concept should be applied in disputed cases.

So why not use conceptual analysis to clarify how disease, illness and sickness are related? The problem is that it is very doubtful that it is possible to uncover standard definitions of disputed health concepts (Hofmann 2001; Knobe & Nichols 2008; Nordby 2006, 2008). The fact that there have been so many unsuccessful attempts to define disease, illness and sickness suggests that there are no 'common' definitions that all speakers of our language will defer to (Nordby 2006). Furthermore, there are deep philosophical reasons for doubting that our common language contains strict definitions of disputed concepts (Quine 1953; Harman 1999; Nordby 2008).

An alternative to looking for general definitions is to define disease, illness and sickness stipulatively. Stipulative definitions are definitions that are assumed to be valid within an area of discourse, like a textbook or an oral presentation. When the application conditions for a concept are defined contextually, the aim is not to capture a general 'common sense' understanding. It is, rather, to use the concept in a way that matches the framework that is defined contextually at the outset.

The problem with stipulative definitions is that contextual concepts cannot have general normative implications (Quine 1953; Harman 1999). A stipulative definition can be useful within the context it is restricted to, but those who have sought to define disease have tried to describe a concept to which all participants in medical discourse, both laymen and professionals, will defer. As Nordenfelt (1987, 8) observes, an analysis that does not capture a common understanding 'would not be used in ordinary discourse, and would therefore be of no interest to us'.

In sum, if we had to use conceptual analyses or stipulative definitions as methodological strategies for exploring whether illness and sickness can be sufficient for disease, the prospects of arriving at substantial conclusions would be bleak. However, it is possible to explore the question of sufficiency in another way. An alternative strategy is to explore the concepts in the light of influential *theories* about health. This strategy will not appeal directly to intuitions about how the concepts apply in 'test cases'. It will instead focus on how the concepts are understood within theoretical perspectives on health and health problems that many have thought of as convincing. Unlike pure conceptual analyses, these theories are not directly grounded in assumptions about 'test cases' in the way Harman explained above.

In fact, this methodological strategy represents a middle course between finding a general intuitive definition and providing a narrow stipulative analysis. The theoretical strategy has a common sense element, in the sense that it invokes theories that many have thought of as convincing. But these theories are grounded in arguments and methodological considerations, not merely in 'pretheoretical intuitions' about how concepts apply.

In the following I employ this strategy. I will appeal to central assumptions within influential theoretical perspectives on the nature of disease. These assumptions will be theory laden, but the relevant theories are theories that many have thought of as plausible. Examining the arguments for these theories falls outside the scope of this chapter. For the present purposes, the important point is simply that they have been very influential. This fact constitutes a good motivation for examining the implications they have.

Evaluative definitions of disease

The theoretical perspectives on disease can be divided into two main camps, evaluationism and naturalism. Evaluationsists hold that the concept of disease refers to health problems that are negatively evaluated as pathological disorders. A well-known proponent of this idea is Fulford (1989, 2005). He makes a sharp distinction between empirical health issues and the general concept of disease, and argues that

> ... in the future we will indeed know much more about the causes (biological, psychological and social) of human experience and behavior. But this will do nothing to resolve questions about exactly which kinds of experiences and behaviours are negatively evaluated, and, hence, pathological (Fulford et al. 2005, 82).

Evaluationists hold that disease cannot be defined in a physicalistic value-free language. According to evaluationists, disease states do not merit status as diseases in virtue of being physiological, natural states that we can discover. Obviously, we learn more about particular diseases as we gradually learn more about biology and the human body, but this is consistent with the idea that the meaning of the general concept of disease is evaluative. Evaluationists hold that we have a natural disposition to describe some bodily states in negative terms, and that these dispositions determine whether the states in question should be labeled 'disease'. According to evaluationism, disease is partly *created* by our use of value-laden language. Evaluationism about disease is a version of constructivism, the idea that many or all objects and events in the world are mind-dependent.[1]

Within this general evaluationist framework, there have been many different attempts to define disease (Lindstrøm 2009). One source of disagreement concerns the scope of evaluative judgments. Are all speakers of our language entitled to determine what disease is, or should some subgroup of 'experts' decide? Another controversial issue concerns the nature of evaluative vocabulary. Some evaluations have accepted that we need a full-blown ethical vocabulary to capture disease. Others have thought that a weaker normative vocabulary is sufficient (Hofmann 2001).

For our purposes here , these differences do not matter. The important point is that evaluationists have focused on traditional pathological conditions when they have discussed the nature of disease. Evaluationists have, in fact, made a sharp distinction between disease and illness. Fulford writes that illness is a concept that

> ... is associated naturally with the patient's experience of ill-health: It is subjective and value-laden, a matter of feelings and sensations, of complaints, and of symptoms (Fulford 1999, 171).

This corresponds to a widespread view: Since disease is a pathological condition – an 'objective' disorder that can be studied in an intersubjective way – an elucidation of the phenomenological concepts of illness cannot capture the nature of disease.

Now, the fact that evaluationists have made this assumption does not mean that it is true. In order to understand whether it is justified, it is necessary to focus on the reasons evaluationists would give for accepting it. Their

---

[1] There can be strong and weak versions of constructivism. A strong version holds that there are no external objects that are mind-independent. This is classical idealism. Weaker versions hold that only some objects are mind-dependent.

main argument is not difficult to understand. According to evaluationists, disease and illness are metaphysical states with entirely different properties. Evaluationists have therefore assumed that the project of defining disease is radically different from the project of defining illness. But is this really so?

I think the reason why this question has not received much attention can be traced to the idea of conceptual analysis, as I described it above. For those who have attempted to define disease, the key question has been whether a suggested definition matches the pretheoretical intuitions we have about paradigm cases of disease. That is, cancer, aids, arthritis, and other typical cases of disease must fall under the definition, while typical cases of pathological disorder that are not diseases – states like injuries – should not fall under the definition (Nordby 2006). The reason why evaluationists have not dealt with states of illness is simply that these states have fallen outside the intended scope of the analysis of disease. They have not been thought of as relevant to the process of evaluating definitions of disease.

However, it is not *a priori* obvious that an evaluationist analysis of disease cannot be used to capture illness. In fact, it seems that there is nothing in principle that should prevent an evaluationist from inflating the scope of his definition. Consider a state like pain, the paradigm example of illness. Why not suppose that this can be negatively evaluated in the same way as a somatic disorder of disease? It seems that it is perfectly acceptable for evaluationists to hold that pain states qualify as diseases as long as they are evaluated negatively.

The point becomes even clearer if we consider combinations of illness and sickness – the typical grey cases of long-term sickness absence (chapter 5). In these cases, the label 'sickness' is normally regarded as a negative label, in the sense that it is often conceived to be 'not good' or 'bad' for a person to be absent from work. The evaluationist analysis applies, and the evaluationist can accept that illness and sickness are jointly sufficient for disease.

This is not necessarily meant as a critique of evaluationism *per se*. It is possible to be an evaluationist and accept, already from the outset, that illness and sickness can be sufficient for disease. The point is that this is not how evaluationism traditionally has been understood. The fact that it is possible for an evaluationist to accept that illness and sickness are sufficient for disease, constitutes a challenge for the *standard* but not necessarily only conception of evaluationism. This means that evaluationists who think that we should make a fundamental distinction between illness, disease and sickness must give a more robust argument for why we should make such a distinction. Evaluationism, as an 'ism', does not allow us to make a sharp distinction.

Naturalism and the harmful dysfunction analysis of disease

The other main tradition in the debate about the nature of disease is naturalism. Naturalism is the view that disease states can be described in naturalistic and scientific terms (Nordby 2006). According to naturalists, states of disease are real states in the world - states that can be discovered and studied just like everyday natural objects and events in the world around us. As Lindstrøm notes, the key concept in naturalism is realism:

> Underpinning naturalism is typically a firm conviction that diseases somehow are objective patterns in the world, which medical ... and life scientists can discover by employing conventional scientific-empirical methods (Lindstrøm 2009, 13).[2]

There are different schools within naturalism. A main dividing line can be drawn between those who think that disease states can be understood and described intrinsically, and those who think that they have to be explained functionally.[3] Function, in turn, has been understood in different ways. It has been understood causally in a strict physiological sense, and biostatistically in a less physicalistic sense (Hofmann 2002; Boorse 1997).

Like evaluationists, naturalists have focused on traditional diseases. But this does not mean that it is *a priori* impossible to use the naturalistic framework to analyze illness. So what happens if we employ the naturalistic perspective when a person experiences illness and has a sickness certificate? Is it possible for naturalists to accept that this can be sufficient for having disease?

This question does not have a straightforward answer. The reason is that naturalists will disagree about certain fundamental assumptions. It is difficult to explore any substantial *general* consequences of naturalism. There are,

---

[2] Naturalism is a version of (metaphysical) realism, the idea that many concepts refer to objects and events in a mind-independent external world.

[3] According to a functional explanation, the nature of a state or event can be understood by understanding the role the state or event has in networks. Networks, in turn, are often understood as causal networks.

however, some naturalistic theories that have received more attention than others. These theories have been thought of as paradigm theories, and their implications are therefore particularly interesting since many naturalists will accept them. Here I will focus on one of these paradigm theories, namely Jerome Wakefield's harmful dysfunction analysis of disease. Wakefield describes this analysis as

> ... a hybrid account of disorder as harmful dysfunctions, wherein dysfunction is a scientific and factual term based on evolutionary biology ... and harmful is a value term referring to the consequences that occur to the person because of the dysfunction and are deemed negative by socio-cultural standards (Wakefield 1992, 374).

This analysis differs from evaluationism in the sense that the dysfunctional element is a purely naturalistic concept. The reason Wakefield's analysis is not a value-free position is that it requires that the dysfunction is harmful for the individual. For Wakefield, this evaluative concept of harmfulness is first and foremost understood as a biological concept. An organism can function in good or bad ways compared to biological norms for that organism, and it can therefore have a dysfunction that is negative in light of those norms.[4]

However, once it is accepted that evaluative vocabulary is needed to capture disease, there is no reason why the evaluative vocabulary should be restricted to non-ethical evaluative vocabulary. For Wakefield, what is important is the idea that judgments about harmfulness (or non-harmfulness) are needed to capture disease: Less important is how these judgments are based in normative linguistic practices (Wakefield 2005).

This point is highly relevant for understanding whether illness and sickness can be sufficient for disease. The reason is that sickness is a sociological norm. Obviously, absentees might think of 'sickness' as a positive label, but this does not happen very often. Persons certified as sick often think of sickness as 'harmful' for psychological, functional, and practical reasons. From their individual perspectives, having a sickness normally affects their experienced quality of life, their ability to work, and their desire to live their lives in the way they endorse.[5] Furthermore, these subjective experiences normally

---

[4] Wakefield has pointed out in conversation that he is inclined to accept an Aristotelian 'teleological' concept of function.
[5] This point is discussed in many other chapters in this book.

correspond to external perspectives. From the perspectives of absentees' doctors, social workers, workplaces, and the society as a whole, sickness absence is usually evaluated negatively for economic and other reasons.

The upshot of this is clear. First, long-lasting illness that leads to sickness absence can be regarded as a dysfunction compared to medical norms, experienced well-being, and functional abilities. For instance, having severe chronic headache is to be in an inner medical state that elicits a significant negative first-person experience – things are not working smoothly within the body. Long-lasting pain involves a negative biological 'friction', a deviation from a medical standard. In the most fundamental sense, a bodily process is not functioning in a way that corresponds to norms for how it should function.[6]

Second, when a state of illness leads to sickness, then, as I have just argued, it will normally be harmful, in the sense that it will negatively influence personal well-being and preferred ways of living. It therefore follows from Wakefield's harmful dysfunction analysis that illness and sickness can be sufficient for disease.

Remember that the argument did not require that illness and sickness *have* to be sufficient for disease. The traditional idea was that the phenomenological nature of illness can never be sufficient for disease – not even when combined with the sickness role. It has standardly been thought that a social sick *role* cannot turn an illness into a disease. I have shown that this is not an inference that the dominant version of naturalism allows us to make. If we apply Wakefield's definition of disease, then we should accept, contrary to what most theorists have assumed, that illness and sickness can be sufficient for disease.

It is important to note that this is a conclusion about principles. In fact, one counterexample would be enough to undermine the general assumption that illness and sickness can never be sufficient for disease. I have argued that there are clearly many counterexamples. Illness can often be conceived of as a dysfunction, and when illness leads to sickness absence, it is usually harmful for the individual.

---

[6] This process can be described on different levels. Wakefield often uses the software-hardware metaphor to explain how he thinks that a human dysfunction can be described on different levels: Sometimes the problem can be described on a software level, and sometimes a physicalistic language and a focus on the hardware level is required.

A modified analysis

What if we take away the 'harmful' part of Wakefield's analysis? As shown, Wakefield admits that his analysis of disease is a hybrid account, in the sense that it contains the condition of harmfulness in addition to the idea of a dysfunction. The reason he includes this condition is that he thinks biological dysfunctions alone cannot be sufficient for disease. As an example he considers is a person who gets much older than normal. This can involve a biological dysfunction, but such a dysfunction is not, Wakefield maintains, a disease in any intuitive sense. According to Wakefield, the condition of harmfulness is needed to exclude this and other counterexamples to a pure dysfunctional analysis. A biological dysfunction can be good or bad for a person, and when it is not harmful, Wakefield claims that it is not a disease (Wakefield 2005).

However, one might think that the clause about harmfulness makes the definition too narrow. Lindstrøm has recently pointed out that Wakefield's definition excludes all organisms that can have disorders that are not harmful (Lindstrøm 2009). But these organisms, Lindstrøm holds, can also be in pathological disease states. Referring to the idea of conceptual analysis as described above, Lindstrøm claims that 'nobody beats Wakefield when it comes to intuition pumping as long as the scope of conceptual analysis is restricted to disorders in humans' (Lindstrøm 2009, 82). But the scope of the definition should be wider: 'The concept of pathology is bound to be bent in a pure naturalistic direction to the extent pathology is predicated of all living organisms' (Lindstrøm 2009, 51).

Lindstrøm argues that if we stick to a pure dysfunctional account of disease, we are able to incorporate all dysfunctions:

> As long as the practical and clinical divisions of medicine do not suffer from this conceptual development, I believe that it is most reasonable to opt for a pure dysfunction analysis of pathology. Such an account may fail to please all the intuitions we hold in our own case, but it will apply to every other species that lives and has ever lived. As it were, we find ourselves being outnumbered a million to one (Lindstrøm 2009, 103).

Lindstrøm calls this the 'million to one argument'. The idea is that Wakefield's analysis more or less matches the intuitions we – as one species - have about ourselves. But there is no room for harmfulness in the case of the millions of other species that can have pathological disorders that are not harmful.

Wakefield could respond to this argument in several ways. One strategy is to argue that dysfunctions can be harmful in organisms other than humans. Another is to argue that dysfunctions in other organisms are not really pathological disorders. In my view, a third option is the best response. What Wakefield should do is to restrict his analysis of disease to organisms that can have subjective experiences. By modifying the analysis in this way, it is possible to meet the challenge from the 'million to one argument'. The aim is not to capture all kinds of disorders, but to identify pathological disorders that it is possible to feel and experience as health problems.

However, the consequence of this strategy is that it becomes even clearer that illness and sickness can be sufficient for disease. For now the analysis explicitly connects disease to subjective experience. In fact, the modified analysis clearly belongs in a comprehensive nursing tradition that ties disease to actual or potential 'psychopathological phenomena' (Carrieri-Kohlman et al. 2005). Thus, restricting the definition of disease to organisms that can have subjective experiences makes it even clearer that the 'dysfunction' definition of disease implies that illness and sickness can be sufficient for disease.

Implications

Where does this leave us? In the philosophical literature on health and sickness, it has often been assumed that absentees' experiences of being ill cannot be sufficient for having 'real diseases'. I have argued that the two dominant perspectives on the nature of disease are inconsistent with this assumption. According to evaluationism, controversial cases of illness and sickness can clearly be evaluated negatively and hence be sufficient for disease. According to Wakefield's naturalistic dysfunctional analysis of disease, a state of illness can involve a dysfunction, and having a sickness certificate can certainly be harmful for an absentee.

Obviously, the idea that illness and sickness can be sufficient for disease does not imply that illness is disease. However, the fact that the theoretical perspectives that I have focused on imply that there can be a relation of sufficiency means that questions about the nature of the three concepts are deep philosophical questions. It is far from clear that we are entitled to make a sharp distinction between disease, illness and sickness.

This conclusion has several dimensions. In the most fundamental sense, it implies that some widespread assumptions about 'grey' cases of illness and sickness absence should be reconsidered. In discussions of long-term sickness absence, it is often held that the word 'disease' can only apply if absentees are in 'medical' states of ill-health that can be 'measured' and 'studied' in an intersubjective, objective way. Some theorists and practitioners have gone one further step and assumed, implicitly or explicitly, that if absentees are not in such objective states, then they are, strictly speaking, not 'really ill'.

These arguments have a positivistic undertone, and they are often associated with the contention that sickness absence that does not involve documented disease is a very problematic category. The analyses of disease that I have presented imply that this contention is problematic. As Hofmann notes above (chapter 2), the traditional idea has been that disease represents the medical profession's perspective on health problems. It follows from both evaluationism and Wakefield's naturalistic analysis that illness should fall under the medical profession's perspective on disease.

What, then, about the nature of disease? Philosophers have often assumed that disease is fully independent of illness (Nordby 2006; Lindstrøm 2009). The idea has been that having disease must involve more than having a negative subjective experience of not being healthy. If illness and sickness absence can be sufficient for disease, then this idea is false. This does not necessarily mean that illness and disease are identical states. After all, identity involves more than sufficiency.[7] However, when one state or event is sufficient for another state or event, then a closer look at the question of identity is merited. Sufficiency is *prima facie* a candidate for identity unless there are independent good reasons for making an ontological distinction (Johnston 1992).

The question of the nature of disease is a metaphysical question – it is a question about how the world is (Nagel 1986). Another question is how we should think and talk about disease states as part of the world. Answers to the metaphysical question have consequences on the level of thought. If we know what disease is, then we know the extension of the concept we should

---

[7] In fact, illness and sickness could in principle constitute disease without being identical to disease. The reason is that constitution is not necessarily identity (Johnston 1992).

use to think about disease. The argument that an absentee's illness can be sufficient for disease is therefore relevant in professional communication with absentees. It is far from clear that doctors and social workers are entitled to make a sharp distinction between the meaning of the expressions 'disease' and 'illness'.[8]

This point is not merely relevant for analyses of doctor-patient interaction and dialogues with absentees. It is also relevant in discussions of how absentees are entitled to think of themselves and their ability to come back to work. Absentees' conceptions of themselves as sick persons can be shaped by theoretical considerations. If the idea that illness can be sufficient for disease is communicated to the public, it could influence absentees' beliefs about their health problems. In fact, the idea could also confirm and strengthen health values and pretheoretical ideologies that already exist. It has been well documented that many patients assume that the meaning of 'illness' is not very different from the meaning of 'disease' (Smith 2002). The problem in doctor-patient communication has been that this assumption does not match the understanding many doctors have (Nordby 2008). If illness can be sufficient for disease, the tables would be turned. It would be patients who have the 'theory' on their side.

Some might think that if absentees form such an understanding of the theoretical relation between illness and disease, then this will influence their motivation for coming back to work in a negative way. Would not the label 'disease' contribute to confirm passivism and absentees' beliefs that they are not able to work? However, this is far from obvious. If a person is absent from work due to illness, she will not necessarily experience her situation as worse if she starts to think that the label 'disease' applies to her.

In fact, it is not unreasonable to assume that the label would make it easier for many absentees to accept their roles as persons with sickness. Instead of focusing on experienced conflicts of meaning and whether they have a 'real disease', they could use their energy to focus on sources of motivation and job-related arrangements, in accordance with a salutogenic approach to health (chapter 12). It is well documented that persons who are absent from work due to illness spend a lot of time reflecting on frustrating experiences

---

[8] I am not claiming that they often make a sharp distinction. The point is, rather, that some might make a sharp distinction, and the arguments in this chapter imply that this would be unjustified.

and on their status as persons who are not working. If it were acknowledged that they have disease, then they could focus on more positive and practical issues – how to live and work as well as realistically possible in the situation they are in.

Conclusion

The assumption that illness and sickness cannot be sufficient for disease has been a presupposition, not an implication derived from substantial analyses. I have explored the implications of two dominant definitions of disease and argued that these definitions imply that the insufficiency assumption is unjustified. And it is the definitions that matter, it is the fundamental definitions that are supposed to tell us what disease really is.

Evaluationists and naturalists might try to revise their analyses in order to make a sharper distinction between disease and illness. But why? There are no *a priori* truths about these relations of conceptual meaning. In fact, following the recommendations of the existing definitions gives us a fresh way of thinking about illness, disease and sickness absence. This way of thinking could change some stubborn ideologies, reduce passivism, and give absentees more positive and action-orientated thoughts about their roles as sick persons. In the end, the focus would be not so much on the label 'disease', but on how it is possible to achieve a sense of coherence and live one's life as well as realistically possible.

References

Baillie, L. 2005. *Developing practical nursing skills.* London, Hodder Arnold
Carel, H. 2008. *Illness.* Stocksfield, Acumen
Boorse, C. 1997. 'A rebuttal on health'. Humber, J. & Almeder, R. eds.:
 What is Disease? Totowa, New Jersey, Humana
Dahlberg, K., N. Drew & M. Nyström 2001. *Reflective lifeworld research.*
 Lund, Studentlitteratur
Carrieri-Kohlman, V., Lindsey, A. & West, C. 2003. *Pathophysiological*
 phenomena in nursing. St Louis, Saunders
Fulford, K. 1989. *Moral theory and medical practice.* Cambridge, Cambridge
 University Press

Fulford, K. 1999. 'Analytic philosophy, brain science, and the concept of disorder'. Chodoff, P. & Green, S. eds.: *Psychiatric ethics*. Oxford, Oxford University Press

Fulford, K. 2005. 'Looking with both eyes open: fact and value in psychiatric diagnosis'. *World psychiatry*, 78–86

Harman, G. 1999. *Reasoning, meaning and mind*. Oxford, Oxford University Press

Hofmann, B. 2001. 'Complexity of the concept of disease as shown through rival theoretical frameworks.' *Theoretical medicine and bioethics*, 211–37

Johnston, M. 1992. 'Constitution is not identity'. *Mind*, 89–106

Knobe, J. & Nichols, S. eds. 2008. *Experimental philosophy*. Oxford, Oxford University Press

Lindstrøm, J. 2009. *Carving mental disorder at the joints*. D.Phil dissertation. The University of Oslo, Department of philosophy

Nagel, T. 1986. *The view from nowhere*. Oxford, Oxford University Press

Nordby, H. 2004. 'Concept possession and incorrect understanding'. *Philosophical explorations*, 54–69

Nordby, H. 2006. 'The analytic-synthetic distinction and conceptual analyses of basic health concepts'. *Medicine, health care and philosophy*, 169–80

Nordby, H. 2008. 'Medical explanations and lay conceptions of disease and illness in doctor-patient interaction'. *Theoretical medicine and bioethics*, 357–70

Nordenfelt, L. & Twaddle, A. 1993. 'Disease, illness and sickness: Three central concepts in the theory of health'. *Studies on health and society*. Linköping, Linköping University Press

Nordenfelt, L. 1987. *On the nature of health*. Dordrecht/Boston/London, Kluwer Academic Publishers

Nordenfelt, L. 1993.' On the relevance and importance of the notion of disease'. *Theoretical medicine*, 15–26

Nordenfelt, L. 2001. *Health, science and ordinary language*. Amsterdam/New York, Rodopi

Quine, W.V. 1953. *From a logical point of view*. Cambridge, MA, Harvard University Press

Reiso, H. 2004. *Work ability and sickness absence: A follow-up study in general practice*. D.Phil dissertation, The Faculty of Medicine, The University of Oslo

Smith, R. 2002. 'In search for non-disease'. *BMJ* (bjm.com), April 2002

Tellnes, G. 1989. 'Sickness certification in general practice: A review'. *Family practice*, 58–65

Wakefield, J.1992. 'The concept of mental disorder'. *American psychologist*, 373–88

Wakefield, J. 2005. 'On winking at the facts, and losing one's hare: Value pluralism and the harmful dysfunction analysis'. *World psychiatry*, 88–89

Østerås, N. 2009. *Functional assessments: A study of functional ability in a population, and structured assessments in general practice.* D.Phil dissertation. The Faculty of Medicine, The University of Oslo

Chapter 8

Social bonds, emotional processes and mental ill-health

Ulla-Britt Eriksson, Bengt Starrin,
Lena Ede & Staffan Janson

Summary

The development of the sickness absence rate in Sweden, with a growing number of diagnoses due to stress, cannot be explained solely by organizational changes. Lately, research on the role of emotions in this context has garnered increasing attention, contributing to our understanding of how external circumstances can influence internal conditions and of how ill-health can develop. Emotions, particularly, the emotion of shame, seem to play an important role. The shame emotion can be described as a primary emotion of great importance for social interaction – as a marker of insecure social bonds. The shame emotion can also be linked to and a marker of the individual's social status. With the changes in the Swedish sickness absence rate as a background, emotion research and theories of sickness are presented in this chapter. An exposition of the concept of shame in social science is given. Even though our knowledge of the frequency of shaming, for example, in the workplace, is limited, there are studies indicating that it is rather common. Having been condescended seems to be strongly associated with long term sickness absence due to mental diagnoses. Finally, the hypothesis of the Burnout staircase, based on an interview study with persons on sick leave, is presented. This hypothesis describes a step-wise process towards sickness absence due to burnout.

Introduction

In the late 1990s, against a background of a dramatic rise in the number of those on sick leave in Sweden, there was an increasing interest in research on sickness absence and its causes. In order to understand the processes leading to ill-health, we will examine in some detail theories on emotions and mental ill-health. We will consider the most cutting-edge research in this field and present some of the more recent studies.

First, we will comment briefly on developments in sickness absence in Sweden during recent decades and draw some parallels with other countries. Since the 1980s, sickness absence has shown considerable fluctuation and dramatic swings (Voss 2002; Lidwall & Skogman Thoursie 2000a; 2000b). A dramatic rise occurred from the late 1990s until 2003, when, in just a few years, the number on sick leave more than doubled and reached its highest level since the introduction of modern health insurance. A wide range of measures were adopted to reduce the number of sickness absences. Since 2003, the level has fallen just as dramatically. Internationally, Sweden is usually compared with eight European countries considered to have comparable health insurance systems. The most recent comparison shows that sickness absence in Sweden among employees aged 20–64 in 2007 was three percent, which is lower than in Norway (3.9%), the country in Europe with the highest sickness absence. Sweden's rate was somewhat higher than Finland's (2.6%) and Denmark's (2.5%) (Försäkringskassan [Swedish National Insurance Office] 2009). The prognosis for 2009 showed a continued decline in Sweden, with sickness absence approaching 2.2 percent, which has been the average level in the rest of Western Europe for the last 20 years (Dutrieux 2010).

During the second half of the 1990s and the early years of the 21st century, long-term sickness absence increased at a greater rate among women than among men. Women on sick leave are also on average younger than men, even though the average age among women on sick leave increased from 43 to 45 between 2003 and 2006. The average age among men increased in the same period from 46 to 47 (Försäkringskassan 2007). The increase in sickness absences which commenced in the late 1990s covered all diagnoses, but a particular increase was noted in mental diagnoses (Palmer 2004; Eklund, Johansson & Sundén 2002). For women, it is mental diagnoses that are most common among those on long-term sick leave. For men, it is the second most common diagnosis after musculoskeletal diagnoses.

Mental diagnoses constitute generally about 25–30 percent of the total number of the long-term sickness absences in Sweden (Lidwall, Marklund & Skogman Thoursie 2004). The mental ill-health diagnoses seem to be increasing in Europe (Järvisalo et al. 2005), and there are global trends towards increasing stress and ill-health at work (Dollard et al. 2007).

Emotions, shame and mental ill-health

Several of the scientific explanations of sickness absence point to shortcomings in the work environment. Psychosocial explanations place great emphasis on the stress that individuals may be exposed to at work or during their leisure time. There are several theories on stress but, in their more general form, it is assumed that external pressures which generate a sense of danger or threat may lead to negative stress. This, in its turn, may give rise to both physical and mental ill-health. Among other things, stress involves emotional strain. Richard Lazarus, an American stress researcher, makes it very clear that stress, emotions, and coping, i.e. how one handles stress, are linked (Lazarus 1999). The three concepts form a conceptual unity, in which emotions are superordinate, since they include both stress and coping. Separating them is only justified for analytical purposes. Lazarus maintains that it is very reasonable to assume a link between stress emotions and certain illnesses. At the same time, he points out that we know far too little today about the psychological and physiological mechanisms surrounding these links.

Thus, there is a lack of knowledge regarding the specific emotions which accompany stress and which can generate illness. It is possible that research on the form of stress that threatens self-esteem is a significant piece of the puzzle. In a number of studies, an American research team has shown that, if the threat or danger includes an evaluative component leading to a deterioration of one's self-image, stress may have serious effects on health. What is at stake here is the potential risk that other people may view the individual in negative terms. Research carried out by Sally Dickerson and her team suggests this connection (Dickerson, Gruenewald & Kemeny 2004). They focus on shame as a key response when the social self is threatened. This happens, for instance, when, an individual is rejected, loses respect, loses face, or feels he or she is a failure and of lesser value, in short, when one's status has been diminished. When self-esteem is threatened, this, it would seem, does not merely entail running the risk of a range of mental problems. Dickerson and her team have also shown that, in cases of acute threat to the social self, there is increased production of cytokines (Gruenewald, Dickerson & Kemeny 2007). Cytokines indicate that an inflammatory process may be in progress. It would seem, therefore, that people are very anxious and worried about being faced with new tasks or situations which involve an evaluative component directed at the self. We are highly motivated to maintain self-esteem, and we seem to be vigilant in resisting anything that might threaten it.

The German researcher Norbert Semmer (2007) also focuses on the stress that arises when the self is exposed to harassment. Stress as offence to self (SOS) is a broad concept, which considers bullying to be merely one of several types of harassments to which employees may be exposed. Harassment may also involve a rough tone of voice, withholding information, lack of consideration, a poorly functioning ITC system, and having to carry out tasks for which one is not qualified.

In a sense, stress as offence to self offers new perspectives on what stress may entail. But, at the same time, it is old knowledge. It has always seemed self-evident that harassments and humiliations may lead to serious consequences both for the individual and for society. This was apparently the case even during the Viking age, if one accepts that the Icelandic sagas provide a reasonably accurate description of life at that time. The Icelandic sagas contain accounts of life on Iceland during the period 900–1000. They depict a social culture in which the rituals for how an honourable man attains and maintains his honour and esteem are highly regulated. The sagas often discuss the importance of winning respect in one's own eyes and in those of others. It is only when an individual has gained the respect of the other that he is satisfied with himself. The balance in life is disturbed when a person has been humiliated. To restore one's honour and esteem, it is, in most cases, necessary to wreak vengeance; only thereafter is reconciliation possible. Wreaking vengeance – taking revenge – is not perceived as something primitive (Gurevitj 1997).

William Ian Miller (1993) has written about shame in the Icelandic sagas. He believes that it is important to distinguish between the two ways the humiliated and shamed individual may experience the shame: first, as part of an institutionalised system of norms and second, as a consequence of the judgement of other people that he cannot live up to what is expected of a fully moral and respectful individual. The first type of shame, which is combined with anger and indignation, is the shame that an honourable man feels after being challenged and defeated. The second type, which is combined with self-contempt and self-doubt, is the shame an individual feels when he has *not* succeeded in taking revenge, receiving compensation, or achieving reconciliation.

Thus, to avoid the second type of shame, the individual who has been exposed to humiliation by another person must take action to demonstrate to him and to others that he is honourable. If no opportunity for revenge is given and no honourable reconciliation is achieved, time runs out and the individual is dishonoured and his status is greatly reduced. An example of this is the story of Hávard. He lies in bed in an enfeebled state for a whole year. He feels sorrow because his son has been killed and a sense of having failed to gain compensation for his dead son. When a chance of gaining revenge finally occurs after he has spent three more years in bed, his relatives cannot believe their eyes. This decrepit individual is transformed into a powerful and youthful person (Gurevitj 1997). Through this act, he re-establishes respect both in his own eyes and in those of others.

It is significant that Hávard's depression seems, in the first place, to be a result of his lost honour, and, only secondarily, of his sorrow on the death of his son. In the Icelandic sagas, the perceptions of the people surrounding him completely determine how an individual perceives himself. A man's self-esteem is more or less a mechanical reflection of how the group and local community perceive him. That humiliations occur frequently in the Icelandic sagas may perhaps be due to the fact that it is through humiliation that a man has the opportunity to show his dignity. Consequently, it is not a secret that a person has been humiliated. Shame is not taboo; on the contrary, it is a feeling that concerns the community. The culture of honour turns on compensation and/or revenge.

There are other interesting historical examples where honour and esteem play a central role. The historian Christopher Collstedt (2007) provides a detailed description of the culture of honour among Swedish noblemen during the 18th century. Honour and esteem had to be protected, and there was a well-developed sensitivity as to when they were at stake. Disrespectful behaviour in the form of an odd look, a careless word, or someone turning their back could provide sufficient grounds for a duel to the death. Honour was an external attribute that had to be guarded, and there was a high degree of sensitivity. According to Collstedt, the 18th century nobleman lived in a very potent culture of honour, with its own norms to some extent, and taking matters into one's own hands by challenging a person to a duel was the most powerful way to maintain honour among noblemen and soldiers. They did what men in the Icelandic sagas did; they took the law into their own hands. Anyone who did not accept the challenge was a coward.

This culture became a problem for the Swedish state. As early as the end of the 16th century, legal attempts were made to put a stop to duelling. The law was made more severe in the middle of the 17th century. Anyone who killed another person in duel could be sentenced to death, and the person killed was punished by a dishonourable burial without a priest or rites. At the same time, harsh punishment was introduced for defamation, which was a common reason for duels (Collstedt 2007).

The concept of shame in social science

In social science, there is a whole range of representations of the concept of shame. We will, however, limit ourselves to two which are of particular interest in this context. The first concerns how shame should in principle be understood as a primary feeling which is important for the socio-psychological interaction between people. Shame is thus an indicator of the state of the social bonds. The second —the status-bound sense of shame — links shame to the individual's place on society's social 'ladder'. It is an indicator of the individual's social status.

Shame as an indicator of social bonds

Shame, as an important factor in the social interaction between people, is associated with sociologists such as Charles Horton Cooley, George Simmel, Erving Goffman, Suzanne Retzinger and Thomas Scheff. For both Cooley and Simmel, the sense of shame is a feeling of self-observation. This is central for Cooley (1902/1922) in his so-called looking-glass-self thesis, which, in simplified terms, means that shame and pride are feelings that arise as a result of the looking at oneself from the perspective of the other person or, more precisely, from what one believes is the other's perspective. If one believes that the other person has a negative view of oneself, this arouses a sense of shame, and if one judges the other person to have a positive view, this arouses a sense of pride. But, as Simmel (1901/1983) points out, the social distance between people is of major importance here. We are, in reality, nothing in the eyes of a stranger, who is unable even to distinguish us from others because of his or her lack of personal knowledge. Therefore, according to Simmel, the stranger is only able to affect our self-esteem in a more general and undifferentiated manner. Nor does a very close and confidential relationship give rise to shame. With people who are very close to us and who know more or less all about us, a fault, a transgression, or a small mistake does not matter in light of their familiarity. A person who loves us or is attached to us, Simmel claims, does not direct their attention to things that cause shame. It is, therefore, a blessing to have close friends. In Simmel's view of shame, then, both anonymous and intimate relations provide a safeguard. But when relations are neither very close nor very distant but in the middle distance, this safeguard does not work. In this type of relation, mutual categorisation may occur. One individual may be evaluated by the other, and a single piece of negative information may be perceived as a personal expression of his or her nature. Middle-distance relations are thus very much a source of shame. For Simmel, shame is a broad concept which included everything from a slight embarrassment, such as a scarcely visible stain on clothes, to serious moral transgression. The mild form of shame is a matter of embarrassment and the serious form, one of disgrace. Many modern sociologists and other social scientists have adopted this broad view.

Erving Goffman's (1959) major contribution was his demonstration of the central role that avoiding embarrassment and shame plays as a driving force in human behaviour. People, Goffman argues, are desperately worried about the image others have of them, and they try all the time to present themselves in the best possible light in order to avoid shame. His theories develop and bring to life Cooley's ideas about how shame is generated. He also points out that embarrassment arises as a result of a real, expected, or imagined lack of respect, irrespective of how insignificant it might be. Goffman's examples demonstrate how extremely sensitive people are to the level of respect they are shown.

It would be almost 90 years before Cooley's thesis on shame and pride as self-reflecting feelings and as indicators of the state of the social ties between people would be the subject of more detailed consideration and development. Independently of each other, the sociologists Thomas Scheff (1990) and Suzanne Retzinger (1991) have carried out this ground-breaking work. They developed Cooley's ideas on shame and pride as indicators of the state of the social ties between people. People have a need to feel secure, valued, and appreciated by others. Shame signals that this security may be threatened, with the potential risk that one will be socially excluded and rejected and that serious and long drawn-out conflicts may ensue. Pride, by contrast, indicates that there is no problem. Thus, shame signals uncertain and insecure social relations, and pride, certain and secure ones. These feelings may be seen as ingenious signalling systems, like traffic lights for human interaction.

Like Simmel, Scheff advocates a broad definition of shame as a generic term to designate a large group of feelings which arise when individuals see themselves negatively, even if only slightly so, through the eyes of others, or when they expect such a reaction. Scheff's definition includes both less intensive forms of shame, like embarrassment, and more powerful forms, like humiliation, degradation, and disgrace. This may be seen then as a first step towards a scientific definition of shame.

There are many closely related or interchangeable terms for feelings which arise when one sees oneself in negative terms through the eyes of others: for example, feeling 'rejected', 'unworthy', or 'inadequate'. Scheff also discusses the fact that 'too much' esteem, 'too much' consideration and 'too much' respect may also cause shame. Shame arises in this case, then, because one feels that one receives too positive an assessment and far too much in relation to what one thinks one deserves. Thus, praise and the feeling that it is 'too much of a good thing' may be perceived as disturbing social relations, in the sense that there is a lack of harmony which feels embarrassing.

For Scheff, shame is the most dominant feeling because it fulfils more functions than other emotions. First, shame is a key component of consciousness and moral sense. It signals moral transgression even without words or gestures. Shame is our moral gyroscope, so to speak. Second, shame arises in situations where the social bonds are threatened. It is a signal of uncertain and threatening social relations and should therefore be seen as a relational feeling. Third, shame plays an important role in regulating the expression and, indeed, the consciousness of all the other emotions, such as anger, fear, guilt, and love. The extent to which we permit the expression of these emotions depends on the degree to which we are ashamed of them. If one is ashamed of showing anger, then one restrains the feeling. One can be so ashamed of one's feelings that they are completely repressed (Scheff 1990; 2003).

Shame as a regulator has been dealt with in detail by a number of authors, including the German sociologist Norbert Elias and the American historian of ideas Peter Stearns. The sense of shame for which Norbert Elias (1939/1991) argues in his work on the process of civilisation has both a societal and a private side. He formulates the link between the two more or less as follows. The more the outer constraints from the social structure are transformed into inner self-discipline and self-control and the more extensive the pressure to adapt to prevailing conventions is, the more the fear of transgressing social boundaries or norms is expressed as a sense of shame. Elias' argument is that the history of the process of civilisation is a history of increased emotional self-discipline and self-control. The threshold for what was perceived as embarrassing or shameful was gradually lowered, and one characteristic feature of this is that people exercised increasing self-restraint, self-discipline, and self-control. One of Elias' major contributions in his studies of the process of civilisation was just that he discovered the social significance of shame and the central role that the sense of shame plays in understanding changes in human behaviour.

However, the process of civilisation has a paradoxical consequence in Elias' discussion. On the one hand, it increases people's intertwinement, leading to greater interdependence. On the other, it strengthens people's perceptions of being isolated from each other. The process of civilisation not only places greater demands on the ability to master and control one's own feelings, but it can also do so in a way that leads to more artificial, uncommitted, and indifferent attitudes to other people.

In his book, *American Cool*, Peter Stearns (2004) advances similar ideas. The new emotional culture that emerged concurrently with modern society encouraged a certain degree of emotional passivity in that the embarrassment threshold for intensive feelings was lowered. So-called immature emotional expressions, such as showing anger or envy, should be restrained and corrected with the aid of the sense of embarrassment. Embarrassment was the technique by which reason would replace emotional action without triggering defensive emotional expression.

In modern society, shame and variants of shame, like humiliation, seem to have become increasingly invisible. This is not because they have become less common but because there is something of a taboo against showing others that one is ashamed and humiliated.

Status-bound shame

The second view of shame, which we may term status-bound shame, concerns the link that shame has with low social status, low social class, and social subordination. Even if the sense of shame is an inevitable aspect of human life, status-bound shame focuses on the feeling of being – against one's will – in a subordinate position and in a context where feelings of inferiority thrive. They thrive because shaming is a part of the exercise of power. Causing someone to feel shame signifies having the upper hand. A person who feels shame submits. This idea is found in the works of several of those who have an interest in status-bound shame (see, for instance, DeBotton 2004; Dahlgren & Starrin 2004; Lehtinen 1998; Neckel 1991; Scheff 1990).

In his work *Status und Scham*, the German sociologist Sighard Neckel (1991) examines the link between the feeling of inferiority and shame. It is typical of the society in which we live that life stories and social circumstances tend to become an individual's personal responsibility. Therefore, conditions such as poverty and unemployment are increasingly experienced as personal defeats.

In western society, there has been a cultural change in people's image of themselves. It is essential to purvey a superior and controlled image in one's personal performance. The search for truth and the search for an authentic self have fallen into the background in favour of the functional self. This functional self is afraid of feeling inferior, and the training of the functional self is geared toward demonstrating that one is superior and pre-eminent in one's personal self-representation. The functional self is expected to be able to perform autonomously in relation to the various social forces in society (Neckel 1991). Personal responsibility is the *sine qua non* for a functional self. The norm is: You shall not be dependent.

For Neckel, both superiority and inferiority are forms of social relation. To feel inferior is to feel that one is worse, less capable, and less competent than others. Inferiority is thus a sense of weakness and incompetence which arises when one compares oneself with others.

One's own achievements are of increasing importance in modern society. Blaming failures on social circumstances is a sign of inferiority. However, to admit that one is ashamed is also a sign of the weakness, which one both despises and feels, must be avoided at all costs. Shame is an emotion that one cannot show, since it is the visible results of having a negative view of oneself. Showing one's shame also reveals the influence of the valuations others have made. This means that, in one's emotional state, one has made oneself dependent on the judgement of others and, consequently, is unable to achieve the desired degree of excellence and autonomy that has become the norm in postmodern society (Neckel 1991).

In modern society, one aspect of shaming involves the public ritual of degradation, for instance, in the institutions of the modern welfare state. Clients on social security must agree to allow their failings to be evaluated in order to qualify for support. To gain access to material resources, then, those seeking social security must give up their self-value, and their chances of defending themselves against the stigma affected by their changed status are limited.

The American sociologist Richard Sennett (1998) takes up the same theme in his book, *The Corrosion of Character*. In it, he examines one of society's major taboos, the fear of failure. One keeps one's failures to oneself. One does not speak about them. As a result, mental fixation and shame increase. Those who suffer most are those who are dependent of society's welfare support, since there is a suspicion that they are parasites and do not really need assistance. Sennett considers the ideology of social parasitism a powerful disciplinary tool. It makes people who are dependent on support from society ashamed. But, as Sennett points out, the sense of failure no longer affects just the poor, the poorly educated, and other exposed groups. The rapid changes in society – globalisation, flexibilisation, and downsizing – make it increasingly common even in the middle class. The feeling of not being good enough and of being inferior to others becomes a sense of shame just because our achievement-oriented culture tells us that our plans will succeed. And when things do not work out as planned, it is easy to accuse oneself, to think and feel 'I am no good, I am worse than the others'. However, as the philosopher

Ullaliina Lehtinen (1998) points out in her doctoral dissertation, *Underdog Shame – Philosophical Essays on Women's Internalization of Inferiority*, the sense of failure and inferiority not only undermines self-esteem and adds to the shame but is also self-destructive. It not only causes self-dissatisfaction but, in the worst case scenario, leads to self-hate. In the encounter with 'superior' people, the shame of subordination may find various forms of expression, such as silence, submissiveness, hesitation, self-doubt, subjection, anger, suspicion, as well as provocative, insolent, and aggressive behaviour. The shame of inferiority and subordination has its basis in a discrimination that is difficult to see and not always intentional. The lack of appreciation shown to people in subordinate positions is a significant cause of reduced self-esteem and self-respect.

How common is shaming?

Information is limited about how frequently people experience being treated in a degrading manner, humiliated, violated, or shamed in some other way. Many maintain that it is more common than is generally believed.

Swedish data suggest that there is a very clear link between humiliation and age. Humiliation diminishes with increasing age (Starrin 2008; Starrin & Wettergren 2010). One explanation might be that people become less sensitive with increasing age or that they become more tactful and considerate with age. However, it might be the case that the older one is, the less inclined one is to admit humiliation. Dennis Smith, an English sociologist, (2003) argues that humiliation and shame and the mechanisms underlying them are among the best-kept secrets in Western organisations and societies. The reason is that we are ashamed of being ashamed, and we do not wish to experience the humiliation that is entailed in admitting our fear of being humiliated. Subtle forms of humiliation and other kinds of shaming occur without becoming visible; this is apparent from the English scientist Tim Kitwood's (1997) study of institutionalised social care of dementia patients. Among the points he discusses are the following psychological principles practised by institutions and care workers: deceit, creating powerlessness, infantilisation, threats and fright, intrigue, stigmatisation, declaring patients incapacitated, banishment, disregard, accusations, derision, and disparagement.

In many workplaces, shame and humiliation seem to be part of the game of social power and intrigue. The American scientist Vincent Waldron (2000) provides detailed descriptions of how this game operates. Public humiliation is used in the struggle for power, position, and authority. Waldron gives the example of Helen, a department head who believed she had the director's ear. During a management meeting where the director presented his plans for the coming financial year, Helen thought there was a mistake in the calculation. She expressed her reservation during the meeting. The director responded with a scornful snort and rejected her reasoning. Helen described how hurt, deflated, and shocked she was at this public reprimand.

Waldron considers public humiliation a form of emotional tyranny which seems to be fairly common. The seriousness of the emotional reactions increases with the distance between the leader and the person humiliated. He says this type of public exclusion is just as painful as receiving a punch in the stomach from a heavyweight boxer.

Organisations – unintentionally or intentionally – use shaming and humiliation as a means of maintaining the desired form of social control. They create scapegoats and thereby transfer the guilt to a victim in a situation where the self-image of the group/organisation might otherwise be threatened and appear in an unacceptable light. Those who sound the alarm, so-called whistle-blowers, are often seen as troublemakers. They are humiliated and risk being completely isolated (Douglas 1995; Pattison 2000). Isolating people from a former fellowship is an effective way to deprive them of their social resources, identity, and group solidarity. Isolation places them in an exposed position and thus makes it possible to manipulate them.

Shame and mental ill-health

Shame is a complex feeling, partly because it has a double nature. On the one hand, shame is a natural and normal aspect of social life. It signals that there is something amiss in the relationship between two people and makes us aware that the social bonds risk coming apart unless something is done to repair them. There is an imperative in shame: 'Dare to admit it'. 'Make an effort to repair the social ties'. The psychiatrist Johan Beck-Friis (2010) says that a person who dares to feel shame and dares to show shame has the feeling of having been thrown off the yoke that is, a real sense of relief. Coming to terms with one's own shame is like discarding the old. However, it requires courage to dare to face shame – above all one's own but that of others as well. It is the unpleasant nature of shame that we fight against, and it takes courage to deal with it. Having this courage and daring to show shame is proof of mental strength. Beck-Friis maintains that this is an important aspect of what we mean by moral courage. Moral courage is a matter of the individual's courage to stand against the bad false self in both oneself and one's surroundings. The capacity for moral courage builds, in part, on the capacity for mature shame.

We are all aware that humour provides relief and may be a means of releasing shame. Humour helps us get through many embarrassing situations. A good laugh can really free us from the shame that disturbs us. Shame emerges into the light and fades away until it finally dissolves (Beck-Friis 2010). However, an evil laugh is a scornful laugh which directed against the other produces reactions of shame in them. The good laugh is not directed against, but rather with, the other or oneself. Laughing at oneself or together with others provides release.

On the other hand, shame can be oppressive, destructive, and excluding and it can result in a series of negative consequences such as mental ill-health. The harmful consequences become more evident when the sense of shame, the feeling of humiliation, is repressed. That may occur if the individual is exposed to repeat shaming which he or she is unable to handle. Studies (Gilbert 2000; Lewis 1987) show that the shame and humiliation involved in personal rejection, public disparagement, personal failure and the like (Kendler et al. 2003; Brown, Tillis & Hepworth 1995; Scheff 2001) may lead to depression. Kenneth Kendler, an American physician, and his collaborators, in a study of the relations between social loss, humiliation, and depression, show that humiliation seems to be as significant a factor in explaining depression as social loss. Further, these factors taken together constitute a tangible risk for severe depression. Still other studies show that the experience of shaming in the form of humiliation is a significant cause of depression (Brown, Tillis & Hepworth 1995) and that shaming co-varies with mental ill-health among those on social assistance (Starrin, Kalander Blomqvist & Janson 2003) and the unemployed (Starrin & Jönsson 2006; Rantakeisu, Starrin & Hagquist 1999).

It would seem that there are two common factors uniting the different forms of depression: a loss of self-respect (Beck-Friis 2010) and insecure social bonds (Scheff 2001). Beck-Friis sees depression as one of several means of mentally defending oneself against shame. Depression is an interruption of mutuality through the withdrawal into oneself resulting from the depressive feeling. An individual with depression is really seeking fellowship but takes responsibility for having caused the break. This acceptance of responsibility and punishment of oneself are typical depressive reactions.

In a study of men in a mental hospital suffering from depression, Scheff (2001) makes the observation that it was characteristic of these men that their social bonds to other people were cut off or very weak. The men showed no sign of either sorrow or anger. Their faces were empty and expressionless. However, they showed what Scheff termed basic indicators of shame, such as the lack of eye contact, slow movement, nervousness, and self-recrimination.

Shame, social bonds and mental ill-health in those on long-term sick leave

In a Swedish study Liv & Hälsa (Life & Health) from 2004, respondents were asked whether, during the three previous months, they had been treated in a degrading manner (Kalander Blomqvist & Janson 2005). As is seen in table 1, examination of the relation between degrading treatment and sick leave for mental health reasons revealed that degrading treatment co-varied with sick leave (lasting longer than 28 days) for mental health reasons. However, we cannot here be certain of cause and effect.

Table 1: Derogatory treatment and long-term sick leave on account of mental disorders including burnout among females (F) and males (M).

	Long-term sick leave longer than 28 days, mental causes	
	F %	M %
Non-derogatory treatment	4	2
Yes, on occasion	7	4
Yes, several times	15	10

The burnout staircase – A description of the burnout process

Previously we have considered the importance of social bonds for our well-being and the role that the emotion of shame may play in the development of ill-health. Shame may be seen as an indicator of threatened social bonds. On the basis of an empirical study, we shall describe the steps towards long-term sick leave for burnout.

The diagnosis 'burnout' attracted much interest in the Swedish debate in connection with the stress-related ill-health patterns that began to be the focus of attention in the late 1990s. In his doctoral dissertation, Friberg (2006) presented the idea that the emergence and popularity of the diagnosis in Sweden was partly due to the fact that it gained legitimacy as a diagnosis when it was included in the medical classification system ICD-10. This occurred in Sweden in 1997. Burnout is not a well-defined concept. It is used in everyday language, in health-care, and as a scientific concept with partially differing meanings (Jenner & Segreaus 1989; Friberg 2006; Starrin, Larsson & Styrborn 1990). In the following study, we are not so much interested in the concept but in its content.

Below we describe the hypothesis of the burnout staircase based on a qualitative interview study. The study was published in 2008 and the description below is a shortened version of previously published material (Eriksson, Starrin & Janson, 2008).

Our aim was to study what caused burnout or such severe stress that it led to long-term sickness absence (lasting longer than 28 days). We interviewed 32 individuals (26 women, 6 men), who were on long-term sick leave with a diagnosis of burnout, and we used grounded theory to analyse the data.

The study revealed a number of critical phases and events relating to the work environment faced by all the participants. In our interpretation, these events represent important phases which contribute to an understanding of the process leading to sick leave. This process can be described as a flight of stairs. We have named it the burnout staircase (see Figure 1). We describe the various steps below.

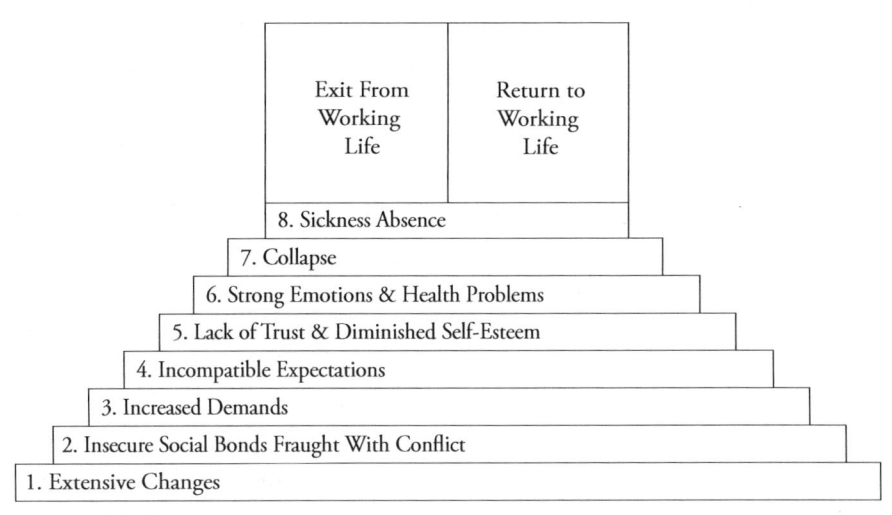

```
               ┌─────────────┬─────────────┐
               │  Exit From  │  Return to  │
               │   Working   │   Working   │
               │     Life    │     Life    │
          ┌────┴─────────────┴─────────────┴────┐
          │         8. Sickness Absence         │
     ┌────┴─────────────────────────────────────┴────┐
     │                 7. Collapse                   │
┌────┴───────────────────────────────────────────────┴────┐
│          6. Strong Emotions & Health Problems           │
├─────────────────────────────────────────────────────────┤
│        5. Lack of Trust & Diminished Self-Esteem        │
├─────────────────────────────────────────────────────────┤
│              4. Incompatible Expectations               │
├─────────────────────────────────────────────────────────┤
│                  3. Increased Demands                   │
├─────────────────────────────────────────────────────────┤
│       2. Insecure Social Bonds Fraught With Conflict    │
├─────────────────────────────────────────────────────────┤
│                  1. Extensive Changes                   │
└─────────────────────────────────────────────────────────┘
```

Figure 1: The burnout staircase.

Extensive changes in the workplace form *the first step* in the burnout staircase. The changes described were of two kinds: organizational changes and cutbacks. Organizational changes primarily involved a new employer, new areas of work, and changes in the decision structure. The participants reported irregular, extensive changes over which they had no control. They had more work to do but fewer opportunities to influence the work situation, which in the long run affected their health situation. 'No one feels good when living in a state of constant changes', as one of the participants put it.

The changes described in step one led to tensions and put pressure on the social bonds; *the second step* in our model is formed by insecure social bonds fraught with conflict. Participants described how their relations with colleagues, as well as with superiors and/or subordinates, deteriorated. Some had experienced severe harassment and bullying. Some of the interviewees reported that they had been treated without respect by a superior. 'It is incredible to stand here as an adult and be scolded like a little child', as one of the participants expressed it. This type of conflict could also involve withholding important information or be neglected. 'I was treated as if I was invisible. It was as if I had never been at the workplace'.

Increased demands form *step three* and were noticeable both at work itself and in the relationships in the workplace. The problems were aggravated by the fact that the increased expectations were often perceived as incompatible.

These contradictory demands form *the fourth step*. The increased demands also made it more difficult to maintain a high level of quality in social contacts. One woman, whose duties included reception work in a health care centre, spoke about a special occasion when, during a four-hour period, she had counted a total of 120 registered patients. She described the situation as follows: 'They are living people I am working with. They are not machines where I can just push a button, receive the charge, and say thank you and next please'.

Cuts and the need to economise combined with staff reductions prevented them from carrying out their work as they wanted to, leading to a sense of inadequacy.

The new expectations fraught with conflict produced emotional stress and affected the participants' trust in others and confidence in themselves, which is *the fifth step* in the burnout staircase.

In *step six*, strong emotions and health problems became increasingly obvious. The participants expressed strong feelings of insufficiency, inferiority, and inadequacy. These expressions can be seen as expressions of feelings of shame. Humiliation and degradation can be turned inward and result in silence, or turned outward in the form of anger and aggression. 'I was so angry', 'lost my temper', '(wanted) to punch my rage out of me' were expressions showing these feelings. Furthermore, the participants began to suffer from various health problems. Tiredness, memory gaps, heart problems, stomach pains, and attacks of dizziness were some of the problems mentioned. Several participants also remembered a general feeling of sadness and crying fits. They also witnessed that they no longer took any pleasure in their work, and one person even went as far as to say that her 'joy of living had disappeared'. At this stage, many of the participants also began to withdraw into themselves. 'In the end it was just me and the work', as one of them said.

The collapse, which all 32 individuals experienced, is *the seventh step*. This collapse, however, expressed itself in different forms. Several individuals described dramatic collapses; some were able to identify triggering factors such as a confrontation at the workplace, while others could not indicate any special event. Suddenly one day, things just stopped. The body or brain ceased to function normally.

The collapse was the beginning of a long period of sickness absence (*step eight*). Sick leave produced mixed feelings with both positive and negative experiences. Even though some saw positive elements in what had happened, they looked upon the sickness absence – being ill – as a failure, as something shameful. Some accused themselves for getting sick and had a bad conscience at having left their job.

Virtually all the participants had been thinking about their return to working life. Some believed they would return in one way or the other, and a few had begun to reduce their level of sickness absence and work part time. Others were convinced that they would never return to work.

The course of events preceding sickness absence might be understood as a process of emotional deprivation, where the individual is gradually emptied of the life-giving emotional energy that is revealed in joy, commitment, and empathy. We describe this process as a flight of stairs, where the various steps describe the different stages in the process (see Figure 1). Our study suggests that the emotional deprivation that characterises the group we examined is, to a significant extent, a result of social processes as well as relational and emotional ones.

Our results support the research literature earlier described. The social bonds of those on sick leave – with colleagues, superiors, and subordinates – had been damaged, and the former showed marked signs of shame, both verbally and nonverbally. These findings support Scheff's and Retzinger's theories of shame.

Emotional deprivation is also associated with Collin's (2003) concept of emotional energy. Successful meetings with people infuse those taking part with energy, while unpleasant meetings have the opposite effect of draining energy. The participants in our study gave numerous examples of how the arenas where a high degree of emotional energy had previously been created no longer existed. The concept of emotional energy corresponds to the meaning Scheff (1990) and Retzinger (1991) attach to the notions of shame and pride. Shame then corresponds to low emotional energy, and pride to high emotional energy.

Scheff and Retzinger distinguish between normal or acknowledged shame and pathological or unacknowledged shame. We suggest that the emotion that conveys the process of emotional deprivation is unacknowledged shame, which, in its turn, has its basis in social relations at the workplace that are insecure and fraught with conflict.

Concluding remarks

In this chapter, we have considered the role that emotions and social bonds may be said to play in the emergence of burnout and other mental illnesses from both a theoretical and an empirical perspective. Against a background where our workplaces have seen a transformation in work from material to relational aspects, greater attention should be paid to emotional work and its effects. Our presentation suggests that social relations and emotions are of considerable importance for an understanding of how illness, mainly mental illness, arises. In chapter 9, aspects of the burnout staircase model are empirically tested.

Acknowledgements

Figure 1 was originally published in *Qualitative Health Research* (Eriksson, Starrin & Janson 2008).

References

Beck-Friis, Johan 2010. *Den nakna skammen.* Stockholm, Natur & Kultur.
Brown George W, Tillis O Harris, & Cathy Hepworth 1995. 'Loss, humiliation and entrapment among women developing depression: a patient and non-patient comparison'. *Psychological Medicine*, 25, 7–21
Collins, Randall 2003. *Interaction ritual chains.* Princeton, NJ, Princeton University Press
Collstedt, Christopher 2007. *Duellanten och rättvisan: duellbrott och synen på manlighet i stormaktsväldets slutskede.* Lund, Sekel bokförlag
Cooley, Charles Horton 1902/1922. *Human Nature and the Social Order.* New York, Scribner's
De Botton, Alain 2004. *Status Anxiety.* London, Penguin books
Dahlgren, Lars & Bengt Starrin 2004. *Emotioner, vardagsliv och samhälle.* Malmö, Liber
Dickerson, Sally S., Gruenewald, Tara J. & Kemeny, Margaret E. 2004. 'When the Social Self Is Threatened. Shame, Physiology and Health'. *Journal of Personality*, 72, 6, 1191–1216

Dollard, Maureen et al. 2007. 'National surveillance of psychosocial risk factors in the workplace: An international overview'. *Work & Stress*, 21, 1–29

Douglas, Tom 1995. *Scapegoats*. London, Routledge

Dutrieux, Jon 2010. Personal communication, 2010–02–12

Eklund, Maria, Birgitta Johansson & Annika Sundén 2002. *Sjukskrivnas syn på hälsa och arbete* (Sickness absentees' view on health and work, in Swedish). Stockholm, Riksförsäkringsverket

Elias, Norbert 1939/1991. *Civilisationsteori del 2. Från svärdet till plikten: samhällets förvandlingar*. Stockholm, Atlantis

Eriksson, Ulla-Britt, Bengt Starrin & Staffan Janson 2008. 'Long-Term Sickness Absence Due to Burnout: Absentees' Experiences'. *Qualitative Health Research*, 18 (5), 620–632

Friberg, Torbjörn 2006. *Diagnosing burn-out: An Anthropological Study of a Social Concept in Sweden*. Lund, Lund University Press, Dissertation

Försäkringskassan 2007. *Långtidssjukskrivna – demografi, arbete, yrke, diagnos, sjukpenningrätt och återgång i arbete 2003, 2005 och 2006*. Försäkringskassan, Försäkringsdivisionen, Enheten för analys, Redovisar 2007:6

Försäkringskassan 2009. *Sjukfrånvaron i Sverige – på väg mot europeiska nivåer? Utvecklingen i åtta länder 1990–2007*. Försäkringskassan, Social Insurance Report 2009:10

Gilbert, Paul 2000. 'The Relationship of Shame, Social Anxiety and Depression. The role of the evaluation of social rank'. *Clinical Psychology and Psychotherapy*, 7, 174–189

Goffman, Erving 1959. *The Presentation of Self in Everyday Life*. Garden City, New York, Doubleday

Gruenewald, Tara L., Dickerson, Sally S., & Kemeny, Margaret E. 2007. 'A social function for self-conscious emotions – the social self preservation theory'. Tracy, Jessica L., Richard W. Robins & June Price Tangney eds.: *The Self- Conscious Emotions. Theory and Research*. New York, The Guilford Press, 68–87

Gurevitj, Aron 1997. *Den svårfångade individen*. Stockholm, Ordfront

Jenner, Håkan & Vera Segraeus eds. 1989. *Att hålla lågan levande: om bemästrande av utbrändhet*. Lund, Studentlitteratur

Järvisalo, Jorma et al. 2005. *Mental disorders as a major challenge in prevention of work disability. Experiences in Finland, Germany, the Netherlands and Sweden*. Helsinki, Finland, Kela, The Social Insurance Institution

Kalander Blomqvist, Marina & Staffan Janson eds. 2005. *Värmlänningarnas liv och hälsa 2004*. Karlstad, Karlstads Universitet, Landstinget i Värmland, Karlstad University Press

Kendler, Kenneth S. et al. 2003. 'Life Event Dimensions of Loss, Humiliation, Entrapment, and Danger in the Prediction of Onsets of Major Depression and Generalized Anxiety'. *Archives of General Psychiatry*, 60, 789–796

Kitwood, Tim 1997. *Dementia Reconsidered*. Backingham, Open University Press

Lazarus, Richard S. 1999. *Stress and Emotion: a new synthesis*. London, Free Association Press

Lehtinen, Ullaliina 1998. *Underdog shame – Philosophical essays on women's internalization of inferiority*. Göteborg, University of Gothenburg, Dissertation

Lewis, Helen 1987. 'Shame – the 'sleeper' in psychopathology'. Lewis H.B. ed.: *The role of shame in symptom formation*. New Jersey, Erlbaum

Lidwall, Ulrik & Peter Skogman Thoursie 2000a. 'Sjukskrivning och förtidspensionering under de senaste decennierna'. Marklund, Staffan ed.: *Arbetsliv och hälsa 2000*. Stockholm, Arbetslivsinstitutet, 91–124

Lidwall, Ulrik & Peter Skogman Thoursie 2000b. *Sjukfrånvaro och förtidspension. RFV Analyserar 2000, 2*. Stockholm, Riksförsäkringsverket

Lidwall, Ulrik, Staffan Marklund & Peter Skogman Thoursie 2004. 'Utvecklingen av sjukfrånvaron i Sverige'. Gustafsson Rolf & Ingvar Lundberg eds.: *Arbetsliv och hälsa 2004* (Worklife and health in Sweden 2004, in Swedish). Stockholm, National Institute for Working Life, 173–193

Miller, William I. 1993. *Humiliation and Other Essays on Honor Social Discomfort and Violence*. Ithaca, Cornell University Press

Neckel, Sighard 1991. *Status und Scham – Zur symbolischen reproduktion sozialer ungleichheit*. Frankfurt, New York, Campus

Palmer, Edward 2004. 'Sjukskrivningen i Sverige – inledande översikt'. Hogstedt, Christer et al. eds.: *Den höga sjukfrånvaron – sanning och konsekvens* (The high sickness absence rate - facts and conclusions, in Swedish). Stockholm, National Public Health Institute, 27–80

Pattison, Stephen 2000. *Shame – Theory, Therapy, Theology*. Cambridge, Cambridge University Press

Rantakeisu, Ulla, Bengt Starrin & Curt Hagquist 1999. 'Financial hardship and shame – A tentative model to understand the social and health effects of unemployment'. *The British Journal of Social Work*, 29, 6, 877–901

Retzinger, Susanne 1991. *Violent Emotions. Shame and Rage in Marital Quarrels.* London, Sage Publications

Scheff, Thomas 1990. *Microsociology. Discourse, Emotion, and Social Structure.* Chicago, The University of Chicago Press

Scheff, Thomas 2001. 'Shame and community: Social components in depression'. *Psychiatry,* 64, 3, 212–224

Scheff, Thomas 2003. 'Shame in Self and Society'. *Symbolic Interaction*, 26(2), 239–262

Semmer, Norbert K. et al. 2007. 'Occupational stress research: The Stress-as-Offense-to-Self'. Houdmont, Jonathan & Scott McIntyre eds.: *Occupational Health Psychology: European Perspectives on Research, Education and Practice,* Vol. 2, 43–60. Avioso S. Pedro, ISMAI

Sennett, Richard 1998. *The Corrosion of Character. The Personal Consequences of Work in the New Capitalism.* New York, Norton

Simmel, George 1901/1983. Zur Psychologie der Scham. In *George Simmel: Schriften zur Soziologie.* Frankfurt a. M., Suhrkamp

Smith, Dennis 2003. *Ledmotiv – idéskrift om ledarskap 2003/1*, 71–81

Starrin, Bengt, Marina Kalander Blomqvist & Staffan Janson 2003. 'Socialbidragstagande och statusbunden skamkänsla – En prövning av ekonomi-sociala bandmodellen'. *Socialvetenskaplig tidskrift,* 10(1), 24–47

Starrin, Bengt, Gerry Larsson & Sven Styrborn 1990. 'A Review and Critique of Psychological Approaches to the Burn-out Phenomenon'. *Scandinavian Journal of Caring Sciences,* 4 (2), 83–91

Starrin, Bengt & Leif Jönsson 2006. 'The finances-shame model and the relation between unemployment and health'. Kieselbach, Thomas et al. eds.: *Unemployment and health.* Brisbane, Australian Academic Press, 75–97

Starrin, Bengt 2008. 'Den förödmjukande skammen och psykisk ohälsa'. Berger, Sune ed.: *Regional utveckling - om produktion, livskvalitet och inflytande.* Karlstad, Karlstad University Press

Starrin, Bengt & Åsa Wettergren 2010. 'The Dynamics of Shame and Psychiatric Ill-Health'. Jackson, Raymond G. ed.: *Psychology of Neuroticism and Shame.* Nova Science Publishers (In press)

Stearns, Peter 1994. *American Cool: Constructing a twentieth-century emotional style.* New York, New York University Press

Waldron, Vincent 2000. 'Relational experiences and emotion at work'. Fineman, S. ed.: *Emotion in organizations.* London, Thousand Oaks, CA, Sage Publications

Voss, Margaretha 2002. *Work and health. Epidemiological studies of sickness absence and mortality with special reference to work environment, factors outside work and unemployment.* Stockholm, Karolinska University Press, Dissertation

II. Empirical part

Chapter 9

Influence of insecure social bonds at work and adverse life events: A comparison between long-term sickness absentees with mental diagnoses and a healthy population

Ulla-Britt Eriksson, Lars-Gunnar Engström, Bengt Starrin & Staffan Janson

Summary

The association between psychosocial work factors and sickness absence with a mental diagnosis was examined in order to test the existence of a previously suggested hypothesis of 'the burnout staircase' (see chapter 8), while adding conflicts and losses in private life into the hypothesis. The burnout staircase describes a seven step process prior to long-term sickness absence starting with reorganizations followed by insecure social bonds affecting the work situation and ultimately health. The study population comprised of 2 521 employed persons (1 397 women, 1 124 men) aged 20–64 years, a sub sample derived from the 2002 National Swedish Survey on Health, Working conditions, Life situation and Sick-listing. Through logistic regression, we analyzed the data to see whether psychosocial work environment and conflicts and losses in private life, either independently or in combination, were more strongly associated to sickness absence with mental diagnoses, as compared to a healthy population. The hypothesis was supported. Reorganization and conflicts at work as well as adverse private life events were associated with increased risk for sickness absence with a mental diagnosis. The burnout staircase described in chapter 8 seems to be a suitable model to describe the sickness absence process with a mental diagnosis, and weak social bonds in private life should be included in the model as well.

Introduction

Long-term sickness absence (LTSA) increased dramatically in Sweden from the late 1990s through to 2003. Since 2003, the sickness absence rate has decreased and was, in 2009, close to the medium rate in some countries in Western Europe with similar social insurance system (Dutrieux 2010). In Sweden, employed women are sickness absent almost twice as often as men (National board of health and welfare 2008). The most common reason for sickness absence among women is mental illness (Palmer 2004; Eklund, Johansson & Sundén 2002). Among men, it is the second most common diagnosis after musculoskeletal diagnoses. The employment rates for women and men in Sweden are comparable, around 80 percent, but the labour market is quite segregated with many women working in the health, care, and service sectors. More than 40 percent of the women are employed in the public sector. Women make up a vast majority, around 90 percent, in some of the occupations in the human service sector, for example, nurses, preschool-teachers, and clerks (Swedish government 2004). Differences in work conditions are said to be one reason behind the higher sickness absence level among women (Dutrieux & Viksten 2004; Persson et al. 2001). A recent study from Stockholm County reported that the health of every fifth woman and every sixth man was at risk due to a stressful work environment (Stockholm County Council 2007). Studies have confirmed the impact of psychosocial working conditions on mental distress and well-being (Van der Doef & Maes 1999; Verhoeven et al. 2003).

Results from earlier studies (Eriksson, Starrin & Janson 2008; Eriksson et al. 2010) have shown that reorganizations leading to weakened social bonds manifested in serious conflicts and insults at the workplace increased the risk of sickness absence due to burnout or other mental disorders. We have named this process the burnout staircase (Eriksson, Starrin & Janson 2008).

The hypothesis of the burnout staircase describes a step-wise process to burnout and sick-listing as starting with extensive changes at the work place, like reorganisations. The assumption was made that administrative steps such as reorganisations did not in themselves have to be problematic. However, when changes are made in such a way that the social bonds at the workplace are weakened, leading to serious conflicts and insults, then they may initiate the process towards sickness absence due to burnout and other mental ill-health. This process may be understood as one of emotional deprivation, whereby the individual is gradually emptied of the life-giving emotional energy revealed in joy, commitment, and empathy. The interpretation of the causes of this process of emotional deprivation was that it began when conflicts which arose as a result of radical changes were not resolved but escalated. In Scheff's (1990) and Retzinger's (1991) emotional and relational theory, the emotion shame signals insecure social bonds. Shame is normal and constructive when it contributes to restoring social bonds, but pathological and destructive when it leads to breaking of these bonds. Normal shame is recognized and acknowledged, whereas pathological shame is suppressed and unacknowledged as shame. It has been suggested that the emotion that conveys the process of emotional deprivation is unacknowledged shame (Eriksson, Starrin & Janson 2008). We have illustrated the process towards sickness absence as a flight of stairs, in which the various steps describe the different stages in the process (ibid.). Extensive changes such as reorganisations make up the first step in the burnout staircase and insecure social bonds fraught with conflict constitute the second step (see figure 1, ch. 8).

In a recent study, the existence of the hypothesis of the burnout staircase was tested in a population of sickness absentees with different diagnoses. The findings suggested that having experienced different steps in the burnout staircase was associated with burnout diagnosis, in accordance with the hypothesis. The study revealed strong and significant associations between experience of the steps studied in the burnout staircase and a burnout diagnosis. This was true for all of the steps studied and both for women and for men. Strong and significant associations were also found between each step studied and other mental diagnoses. The social relations at the work place, especially the quality of these relations, seemed to play a major role in the outcome (Eriksson et al. 2010).

In the present study, we wanted to proceed and test the hypothesis by including a healthy population in addition. This makes it possible to study whether or not the psychosocial working conditions differ between healthy persons and those who become sickness absentees. Further, we want to study the impact of weak social relations in private life on sickness absence. In the previous study, the conflicts studied were limited to the work place. The question is this: do weak social bonds in private life – as well as in the workplace – influence the sickness absence and should these also be included in the burnout staircase model?

Men and women tend to have different types of jobs (Dutrieux & Viksten 2004). They therefore typically have different working conditions and may also value health and work differently. Gender-specific analyses are therefore also needed.

The overall aim of the study was to test the hypothesis of the burnout staircase and to study whether the experience of the first two steps in the staircase concerning reorganisations and conflicts differed between a sickness absent population and a healthy population. A second aim was to include weak social relations in private life in the hypothesis and study the impact of these on sickness absence. A third aim was to study whether or not there were any systematic gender differences in relation to the above associations.

Methods

Sample

The study group is derived from the National Survey on Health, Working Conditions, Life Situation and Sick-listing (RFV-HALS) performed by the National Swedish Insurance Board and Statistics Sweden. The survey was carried out as a postal questionnaire to two samples during May/June 2002. One of the samples was a random sample of individuals who began a sick-listing period from the end of January 2002 and were sick-listed for 15 days or longer. The comparison sample was from the general population.

The response rate was 57.2 percent (6 171 persons) for the sickness absent population and 63 percent (3 160 persons) for the general population. The drop-out rate was in line with what can be expected for postal surveys (Eklund, Johansson & Sundén 2002).

Our study group comprises a subsample of 2 521 employed persons aged 20–64 from these two populations. The analysis includes individuals who were employed at the time of answering the questionnaire, since the risk factor of the psychosocial work climate is relevant mainly for them. Unemployed persons and students were therefore excluded. Also, self-employed persons were excluded. The long-term sickness absentees in the sample were still on sick-leave when they answered the questionnaire and had therefore an ongoing sickness absence period longer than three months. In order to be able to make comparisons, the sample was divided into two groups: one group of long-term sickness absentees with a self reported mental diagnosis including burnout (370 women, 119 men), and one group of healthy persons (1 027 women, 1 005 men). The group with mental diagnoses was selected because the previous study suggested that the burnout staircase was a suitable model to describe the sickness absence due to burnout and other mental diagnoses. Mental diagnoses are one of the main causes of long-term sickness absence for women and men in Sweden and constitute generally about 25–30 percent of the total number of the long term sickness absence (Lidwall, Marklund & Skogman Thoursie 2004). The persons with mental diagnoses in the present study reported that the reasons behind their sick-listing were mental disorders (e.g. melancholia, depression, anxiety), burnout (exhaustion depression) or stress. The healthy population consisted of persons who were working at the time of answering the questionnaire or had been short-term sickness absent less than 15 days. Short-term sick-listed were included in the healthy sample, since short-term illnesses generally cover minor illnesses, like the common cold; further, in studies dealing with the causes behind long-term absence, such people are generally considered to be healthy.

Independent variables

Even though the study was not originally designed to test our hypothesis of the burnout process, it contains questions which are nevertheless suited to test parts of our hypothesis. Since it is a study using cross-sectional data, it is not possible to test the actual stepwise process of the burnout staircase. However, it is possible to examine whether or not individuals have reported experiences corresponding to the different steps.

In the present study, we investigated the experiences of the first two steps in the burnout staircase concerning reorganizations and conflicts. These two steps, which initiate the process, are workplace-related and can be influenced. The following six steps are based on the first two steps. Consequently, we look upon the first two steps as crucial for the whole process.

The first step in the staircase, the starting point of the process, is the experience of organizational changes and staff reductions during the preceding year. One question was posed concerning organizational changes, and one question, concerning staff reductions. The response scale was dichotomized for the purpose of the logistic regression (0 = No such experience; 1 = Yes, experience of organizational changes and/or staff reductions).

The second step concerns experiences of serious conflicts and insults. Two questions were posed: 'Have you during the preceding year experienced a serious conflict at your workplace?' and 'Have you during the preceding year been bullied/insulted?' The response scale of the population of sickness absentees was also dichotomized (0 = No such experience; 1 = Yes, experience of conflict and/or been bullied/insulted).

Since the steps in the burnout staircase mainly represent work-related matters, it is an underlying assumption that the sickness absence is to a large extent work-related. In the present study, we also wanted to include the experiences of conflicts and losses in private life in the analyses. Information on weak social bonds in private life was elicited by a question concerning whether the respondent during the preceding year had been involved in any of five different adverse life events. The events mentioned were (1) a divorce/separation from partner, (2) a serious conflict in the family or (3) with close friend and (4) a death in the family or (5) of a close friend. The responses to all five questions were dichotomized into the following categories: 1 = Yes, have been involved in at least one event and 0 = No.

In order to be able to explore the importance of social bonds in working life, in private life, or combination effects, three models were used. The first model dealt with reorganizations and conflicts *at work* (model 1), the second with reorganizations, conflicts, and losses *in private life* (model 2), and the third model was a combination of model 1 and 2 dealing with reorganizations as well as conflicts and losses *both at work and in private life* (model 3).

Dependent variable and statistical analysis

The sickness absent population of interest for our analyses was employed persons that currently were sick-listed with a mental diagnosis, and from the general population, we drew a subsample of employed persons who were not currently sick-listed or were short-term sick-listed less than 15 days.

Multivariate analyses were performed using a logistic regression on three different models as defined above. The present outcome variable had two values: sickness absent with a mental diagnosis, or healthy. All comparisons were made in relation to the healthy level in order to identify differences in the psychosocial work environment and in life events and to see whether or not psychosocial work environment and life events were more commonly associated with sickness absence due to mental diagnoses. Separate analyses were made for men and women in order to be able to explore the possibility of systematic gender differences. We controlled for age, which can be associated with ill-health and sickness absence. We also controlled for education and employment sector (private or public). In the first model (factors at work), we also controlled for weak social bonds in private life, and in the second model (private life events), we controlled for conflicts at work.

The results are presented as odds ratios (OR) for the association between the independent variables and sickness absentees with mental diagnosis, as compared to healthy cases. 95% confidence intervals were computed (95% CI).

Results

Descriptive characteristics of the study population

Table 1 provides an overview of frequency distributions of the study population in relation to background characteristics for men and women separately.

As can be seen from table 1, there was a larger proportion of sickness absentees with mental diagnoses among men in the age group 50–59 years old, as compared to those in other age groups. Among the women, there were no large age differences between the sickness absent and the healthy persons. Women and especially men with mental diagnoses had university education to a higher degree than the healthy women and men. The dominant employer among the sickness absent women was the municipality sector (48%), while for the female healthy group, there was almost as many employed in the municipality (38%) as in the private (37%) sector. A high proportion of men with mental disorders was employed by public employers (40%), as compared to healthy men (27%).

Table 1: Percentage distribution of sickness absentees with a mental diagnosis and healthy persons in relation to age, education and employer. Women and men are presented separately.

	Women		Men	
(n)	Mental d. (370)	Healthy (1027)	Mental d. (119)	Healthy (1005)
AGECLASS				
20–29	12	18	5	17
30–39	27	27	24	25
40–49	29	24	26	25
50–59	27	27	38	25
60–64	5	5	8	8
	100%	101%	101%	100%
EDUCATION				
- 9 years	13	15	21	23
10–12 years	39	44	34	44
- 3 years univ	22	20	23	15
3 years univ -	26	21	22	18
	100%	100%	100%	100%
EMPLOYER				
State	11	10	15	11
Municipality	48	38	22	12
County council	9	12	3	4
Private	28	37	54	69
Other	4	3	6	5
	100%	100%	100%	100%

Cross-tabulation of independent and dependent variables

Table 2 presents the frequency distribution of step one, reorganization, and step two, conflicts, and their combination, in three models within the two groups, sickness absentees with mental diagnoses and the healthy group.

Table 2: Percentage distribution of the steps reorganization, conflicts and combinations of the two within sickness absentees with mental diagnosis and a healthy group, for three separate models.

	Women		Men	
Model (n)	Mental (370)	Healthy (1027)	Mental (119)	Healthy (1005)
Model 1				
Reorganization and conflicts *at work*	25	15	30	11
No reorganization but conflicts	11	6	9	4
Reorganization but no conflicts	30	37	28	40
No reorganization / no conflicts	34	42	33	45
Total	100%	100%	100%	100%
Model 2 Reorganization at work and conflicts/losses. *In private life*	30	28	20	22
No reorganization but conflicts	27	23	24	20
Reorganization but no conflicts	24	25	38	29
No reorganization / no conflicts	18	25	18	28
Total	99%	101%	100%	99%
Model 3 (*Model 1 + Model 2*) Reorganization and conflicts *At work and in private life*	14	8	13	6
No reorganization but conflicts	8	3	5	2
Reorganization but no conflicts	41	44	45	46
No reorganization / no conflict	37	44	37	46
Total	100%	99%	100%	100%

For sickness absent women and men with a mental disorder, it was 1.5 to 3 times more common to have experienced the combination of reorganization and conflicts at work compared to the healthy women and men (model 1). The sickness absent women and men had experienced conflicts at work without any reorganization twice as often as the healthy women and men. Experience of reorganization but no conflicts were more common among the healthy women and men compared to the sickness absentees as well as experience of neither reorganization nor conflicts.

Model 2 shows a somewhat different pattern. A high proportion (30%) of the women with mental diagnoses had experiences of reorganization at work combined with conflicts and losses in private life, but a high proportion (28%) of the healthy women also had such experiences. Among men with mental diagnoses, experiences of reorganization without conflicts were more common (38%), as compared to the healthy group (29%). A higher proportion of healthy women and men had neither been exposed to reorganizations nor conflicts, as compared to the sickness absent women and men.

When looking at work and private life related events together (model 3), both women and men with mental diagnoses showed around twice as much experience of the combination of reorganization and conflicts and/or losses, as compared to the healthy women and men. Women and men with mental diagnoses had almost three times more experiences of conflicts/losses alone, as compared to the healthy women and men.

Logistic regression

The odds ratios calculated in the logistic regression analyses and presented in table 3 could be described in terms of risk factors for sickness absence. In model 1, it was thereby found that reorganizations and conflicts were significantly associated risk factors of sickness absence due to mental diagnosis for men as well as for women. Having experienced conflicts but no reorganizations was also associated with a significantly increased risk of sickness absence with a mental diagnosis.

In model 2, the experiences of reorganizations and conflicts/losses in private life were analysed. The odds ratios showed that conflicts and losses alone were significantly associated risk factors of sickness absence due to a mental diagnosis for both women and men.

Reorganization and conflicts both at work and in private life (model 3) showed almost identical patterns as in model 1, where only work factors were included.

Reorganizations and conflicts at work (model 1), as well as both at work and in private life (model 3), were associated with sickness absence due to mental diagnosis in the expected way among both sexes. However, reorganizations combined with conflicts/losses in private life (model 2) were not significant risk factors either for women or for men. The odds ratios in the analysis showed that conflicts and/or losses alone gave a significant higher risk in all models in contrast to reorganizations alone. Accordingly, conflicts and/or losses seem to be more important for having a mental diagnosis than reorganizations. Reorganization alone did not seem to have a significant impact on sickness absence due to mental diagnoses.

Table 3: Odds ratios (OR) for being sickness absent with a mental diagnosis in three different models. Women and men are presented separately. 95% confidence interval (CI). Significant odds ratios are presented in bold.

Model -combinations of step 1 +2	Women Mental d. OR (CI)		Men Mental d. OR (CI)	
(Model 1) Reorganization and conflicts *At work*	**2.020**	(1.454–2.805)	**3.421**	(2.053–5.702)
No reorganization but conflicts	**2.379**	(1.516–3.734)	**3.723**	(1.722–8.050)
Reorganization but no conflict	0.934	(0.696–1.253)	0.859	(0.525–1.406)
No reorg / no conflict	1		1	
(Model 2) Reorg at work and conflicts/ losses *In private life*	1.248	(0.871–1.786)	0.938	(0.500–1.8379)
No reorg but conflicts	**1.578**	(1.098–2.266)	**2.062**	(1.122–3.791)
Reorg but no conflict	1.090	(0.750–1.585)	1.485	(0.841–2.619)
No reorg / no conflict	1		1	
(Model 3) Reorg and conflicts *At work and In private life*	**2.098**	(1.407–3.130)	**2.811**	(1.473–5.363)
No reorganization but conflicts	**2.821**	(1.666–4.777)	**3.688**	(1.370–9.929)
Reorganization but No conflict	1.055	(0.808–1.379)	1.111	(0.724–1.706)
No reorg / no conflict	1		1	

We controlled for conflicts and losses in private life in model 1 and conflicts at work in model 2. The expected associations in accordance with the results presented above were found, i.e. a positive association between conflicts and mental diagnoses (data not shown). The background variables controlled for and included in the analysis – age, education and sector of employment – had no additional impact on the odds ratios for the outcome variable (data not shown).

Discussion

In accordance with the hypothesis, we found a strong correlation between sickness absence with a mental diagnosis and the combination of reorganizations and conflicts at work with negative private life events. These results are in line with a study of a Hungarian population, which showed that the most important work factor associated with self-reported health was trouble at work, and more so among men (Kopp et al. 2007). Our results also support those of Göransson and her colleagues (2002), who reported similar outcomes.

Interestingly, the patterns for sickness absentees with a mental diagnosis were similar for men and women in the present study. This finding is in line with a study of predictive factors for long-term sick leave and disability pension, where it was found that life events such as conflicts and losses were strong factors for long-term sick leave and disability pension (Bergh et al. 2007). Though that study did not make separate gender analysis, it was assumed that it was valid for both sexes. However, there are some studies showing gender differences. A Finnish longitudinal population study found that serious life events, such as death or serious illness of a family member, violence, and financial difficulties, were significantly associated with subsequent sickness absence among men (Kivimäki et al. 2002). Allebeck and Mastekaasa (2004) also found stressful life events to be associated with increased sick leave among men. The present study, however, did not include exactly the same life events.

Our results indicate that experience of administrative actions such as reorganisations is not sufficient to explain LTSA due to mental disorders but that if these changes have affected the social relations at the workplace in the form of conflicts, there is a strong association with a mental diagnosis. Conflicts at work thus appear to be essential. Further, if the employee faces conflicts or losses in private life, it may also negatively affect the risk of falling ill. Experiencing reorganisations and conflicts at work, as well as conflicts and losses in private life, has strong associations with a negative health outcome. It may be that conflicts or losses in private life provide a general susceptibility to sickness absence due to mental disorders, if they also are combined with conflicts at work. An association between work conflicts and burnout was also found in studies by Varhama and Björkqvist (2004) and by Fujiwara and colleagues (2003). However in a recent study by Magnusson Hanson and her colleagues (2008), no such association was found. This might have to do with the quality of the social bonds (Scheff 2005). For example, Kendler and his research team (2003) found that humiliating events that directly devalue an individual in an important position were strongly linked to risk for depression or depressive episodes.

The rise of sickness absenteeism in Sweden in the years around 2000 followed dramatic changes in the labour market. In a few years in the 90s, the unemployment rate rose from a few to more than 10 percent. These changes led to changes also in the psychosocial working conditions with both working pace and job insecurity rising. The places where women worked (municipality and county councils) were especially affected and underwent major changes (Persson et al. 2001). In the present study, a high proportion of the long-term sickness absent men with mental diagnoses also worked in the municipality sector, as shown in table 1. The rapid labour market changes make it easier to explain the importance of the influence of the working conditions on the well-being found in the present study.

In Scheff's (1990) and Retzinger's (1991) emotional and relational theory on social bonds, there is an integration of self (emotional reactions) and society (the social bond). For them, both shame and pride are self-reflecting emotions which fulfill a major function in revealing the state of the social bonds between persons. They are arguing that shame plays a crucial role in normal cooperative relationships, as well as in conflicts. If shame and being exposed to shaming causes mental ill-health, it must be by definition toxic. This pathological or toxic shame might be crucial to understanding the link between stressful external circumstances and ill-health (Dickerson, Gruenewald & Kemeny 2004; Scheff 1992; 2001; Wilkinson 1999; 2002; 2005). It deals with our universal need to be a part of a group or community, which is one of the most fundamental human needs (MacDonald & Leary 2005; Scheff 1990). Eisenberger and his research group (2003) describes the fear of risking being abandoned, being excluded, and not forming part of a group as social pain. Our results, with the association between weak social relations and LTSA due to mental diagnoses, support these theories. In the present study, the social bonds at the work places and in the private life of the sickness absent employees with mental disorders had been weakened, and this may have influenced their health. However, the role of weak social relations and shame in developing mental illness must be further explored in future studies.

There are a number of limitations to the study. One limitation is that the national survey used for the study was not originally designed to test our hypothesis of the burnout staircase. Further, our findings were based on cross-sectional data, which means that the casual direction of the relationships between reorganizations and conflicts or losses cannot be established. Another limitation with the cross-sectional design is that it prevents us from studying the actual process of the burnout staircase. In this self-reported survey a potential recall bias might have affected especially the sickness absent respondents since they were asked about conditions one year prior to the sick-listing. The methodological strength lies in that the study is based on a large representative sample of the Swedish sickness absentees and the general population. Since our results refer to employed men and women in Sweden, it cannot immediately be generalized to the whole labour market.

In the present study, we have been able to compare a sickness absent population to a healthy population. In accordance with the hypothesis, a relatively strong association was found between reorganizations and weak social relations at work and being sickness absent with a mental diagnosis. In addition, weak social relations in private life were associated with LTSA due to mental disorders, as were weak social relations both at work and in private life. Sickness absent persons with a mental diagnosis had, to a larger extent than healthy persons, experienced reorganizations at their workplace together with conflicts at work, in addition to conflicts and losses in private life. Our results imply that the burnout staircase described in earlier work (Eriksson, Starrin & Janson 2008; Eriksson et al. 2010) seems to be a suitable model to describe sickness absence with a mental diagnosis. Weak and insecure social bonds in private life should preferably be included in the model of the burnout staircase. More studies are needed to test the hypothesis further. There is also a need for qualitative studies, which pay attention to the total life situation for men and women and on what factors influence health.

Implications

The results from the present study indicate a potential to reduce sickness absence through promoting good working conditions and interventions directed towards the social relations at work. In addition to using sound models for organizing work management, attention should be paid to the quality of the social relations at the workplace, and an adequate conflict resolution style should be promoted. Also, working conditions should preferably be adjusted to the employees' private situation thereby promoting a good balance between labour work and private life.

References

Allebeck, Peter & Mastekaasa, A. 2004. 'Risk factors for sick leave – general studies'. *Scand J Public Health*, 32 (Suppl 63), 49–108

Bergh, H. et al. 2007. 'Predictive factors for long-term sick leave and disability pension among frequent and normal attenders in primary health care over 5 years'. *Public Health*, 121, 25–33

Dickerson, Sally S., Gruenewald, Tara L., & Kemeny, Margaret E. 2004. 'When the social self is threatened: Shame, physiology, and health'. *Journal of Personality*, 72(6), 1190–1216

Dutrieux, Jon & Viksten, A. 2004. *Orsaker till skillnader i kvinnors och mäns sjukskrivningsmönster – en kunskapsöversikt.* (Causes of differences in sickness patterns of women and men. A review. In Swedish). Stockholm, Swedish Social Insurance Agency

Dutrieux, Jon 2010. (uppdatering av tidsserie över sjukfrånvaron, som den mäts i Arbetskraftsundersökningarna; personlig kommunikation 2010–02–12). In swedish

Eisenberger, N.I., Lieberman, M.D. & Williams, K.D. 2003. 'Does rejection hurt? An fMRI study of social exclusion'. *Science*, 302 (5643), 290–292

Eklund, Maria, Johansson, Birgitta & Sundén, Annika 2002. *Sjukskrivnas syn på hälsa och arbete.* (Sickness absentees' view on health and work. In Swedish). Stockholm, Swedish Social Insurance Agency

Eriksson, Ulla-Britt, Starrin, Bengt & Janson, Staffan 2008. 'Longterm Sickness Absence due to Burnout: Absentees' Experiences'. *Qualitative Health Research*, 18, 620–632

Eriksson, Ulla-Britt et al. 2010. Insecure social bonds at work, mental illhealth and sickness absence, *WORK*, in press

Fujiwara, K. et al. 2003. 'Interpersonal conflict, social support, and burnout among home care workers in Japan'. *J Occup Health*, 45(5), 313–320

Göransson, Sara, Aronsson, Gunnar & Melin, Bo 2002. 'Vilja och villkor för återgång i arbete' (Intention and terms for return to work. In Swedish). *En handlingsplan för ökad hälsa i arbetslivet* (Action plan for better working life health. In Swedish), Vol. 2002:5, Socialdepartementet, Stockholm, Fritzes, 101–168

Kendler, Kenneth S. et al. 2003. 'Life Event Dimensions of Loss, Humiliation, Entrapment, and Danger in the Prediction of Onsets of Major Depression and Generalized Anxiety'. *Arch Gen Psychiatry,* 60, 789–796

Kivimäki, M. et al. 2002. 'Death or illness of a family member, violence, interpersonal conflict, and financial difficulties as predictors of sickness absence: longitudinal cohort study on psychological and behavioral links'. *Psychomatic Med,* 64, 817–25

Kopp, M. et al. 2007. 'Work stress and mental health in a changing society'. *European Journal of Public Health,* 18(3), 238–244

Lidwall, Ulrik, Marklund, Staffan & Thoursie, Peter Skogman 2004. 'Utvecklingen av sjukfrånvaron i Sverige' (The development of the sick-listing in Sweden, in Swedish). R.Å. Gustafsson & I. Lundberg eds.: *Arbetsliv och hälsa 2004* (Worklife and health in Sweden 2004, in Swedish). Stockholm, National Institute for Working Life

MacDonald, G. & Leary, M.R. 2005. 'Why does social exclusion hurt? The relationship between social and physical pain'. *Psychological Bulletin,* 131(2), 202–223

Magnusson Hanson, L. et al. 2008. 'Demand, control and social climate as predictors of emotional symptoms in working Swedish men and women'. *Scandinavian Journal of Public Health,* 36, 737–743

National board of health and welfare 2008. *Folkhälsa och sociala förhållanden* (Public health and social conditions, in Swedish). Stockholm, National board of health and welfare

Palmer, Edward 2004. 'Sjukskrivningen i Sverige – inledande översikt' (A review of sick-listing in Sweden, in Swedish). Hogstedt, Christer et al. eds.: *Den höga sjukfrånvaron – sanning och konsekvens* (The high sickness rate – facts and conclusions, in Swedish). Stockholm, Statens folkhälsoinstitut, 27–80

Persson, G. et al. eds. 2001. *Health in Sweden – the National Public Health Report 2001.* Umeå

Retzinger, Susanne 1991. *Violent Emotions. Shame and Rage in Marital Quarrels.* London, Sage Publications

Scheff, Thomas 1990. *Microsociology – discourse, emotion and social structure*. Chicago, The University of Chicago Press

Scheff, Thomas 1992. 'Emotion and illness: Anger, bypassed shame and heart disease'. *Perspectives on Social Problems,* 3, 117–134

Scheff, Thomas 2001. 'Shame and community: Social components in depression'. *Psychiatry: Interpersonnal and Biological Processes,* 64(3), 212–224

Scheff, Thomas 2005. *Toward a New Microsociology: Building on Goffman's Legacy.* Boulder, CO, Paradigm Publishers

Stockholm County Council 2007. *Arbetshälsorapport 2007 (*Work health report 2007, in Swedish). Stockholm, Stockholm County Council

Swedish Government Official Reports, SOU 2004:43, 2004. *Den könsuppdelade arbetsmarknaden* (The gender segregated labour market. In Swedish). Stockholm, Fritzes

Van der Doef, M. & Maes, S. 1999. 'The job demand-control (support) model and psychological well-being: a review of 20 years of empirical research'. *Work & Stress,* 13, 87–114

Varhama, L.M. & Björkqvist, K. 2004. 'Conflicts, workplace bullying and burnout problems among municipal employees'. *Psychol Rep,* 94 (3 Pt 2), 1116–24

Verhoeven, C. et al. 2003. 'Job conditions and wellness/health outcomes in Dutch secondary school teachers'. *Psychol Health,* 18, 473–87

Wilkinson, Richard G. 1999. Health, hierarchy, and social anxiety. *Annals of the New York Academy of Sciences.* 896, 46–83

Wilkinson, Richard G. 2002. 'Putting the picture together: Prosperity, redistribution, health, and welfare'. Marmot, Michael & Richard G. Wilkinson eds.: *Social determinants of health.* Oxford, UK, Oxford University Press

Wilkinson, Richard G. 2005. *The Impact of Inequality. How to make sick societies healthier*. London and New York, Routledge

Chapter 10

The impact of psycho-social work environment on sickness absence: Results from the Swedish Life & Health 2008 Study

Lars-Gunnar Engström & Ulla-Britt Eriksson

Summary

The occupational levels of Swedish women and men are very similar, but the labour market is highly gender segregated with women and men occupying different jobs and working in different sectors. Since the sickness absence rate is much higher for women, we wanted to examine men's and women's psycho-social working conditions in relation to sickness absence by means of Karasek and Theorell's job strain model. The study found a strong relationship between long-term sickness absence and the psycho-social work environment. The study suggests that, as a result of the changing labour market, the psycho-social work environment affects sickness absence in almost all types of jobs and that there may be a decreasing number of 'healthy jobs' in the Swedish labour market.

Introduction

Health at work is one of the target areas of the Swedish national public health policy (Socialdepartementet 2008). It deals with well-being and ability to function during the full length of a working life. Work occupies a great deal of time in an adult's life and fulfills several functions. It gives financial support, as well as a sense of community. Work is also a source of identity and self-esteem. Individuals who are outside the labour market are worse off health-wise than those within it. Numbers from the last Swedish national public health report showed that severe pain is very common among persons with early pension leave, and a lower level of mental well-being is more common among persons outside the labour market, as compared to working persons (Socialstyrelsen 2009). However, most persons of working age have a job, and in this chapter, the emphasis is on work environment factors which are supposed to lead to increasing ill-health in large segments of the population.

The benefit system on the Scandinavian welfare model is based on the principle of protecting the citizen from losing income due to sickness, aging, or unemployment (Esping-Andersen 1990). This system places great importance on wage-earning. We have to bear in mind, though, that sickness absence represents only a small portion of sickness among the population in general. It is limited to persons of working age, who are deemed unable to fulfill their work tasks or are searching for a work due to sickness or injury. Sickness absence is thus linked to the health situation of the individual, but the conditions at the work place and in the labour market also play a role.

In this chapter, using the job strain model developed by Karasek and Theorell (1990), we describe and compare the work conditions from the perspective of the long-term sickness absent population and from that of the general population. In doing so, we present a picture of which work environment factors are important for sickness absence. We will concentrate the discussion below on work environment risk factors, since there have been more studies concerning these factors than studies concerning the health promotion factors at work. Throughout the chapter, our analysis of work environment and sickness absence apply to persons of working age, that is, 18–64 years old. Long-term sickness absence (LTSA) is defined as a sick-leave period of at least 29 days during the last year of our study.

Since the Swedish labour market is characterized by a strong gender segregation with women and men typically in different professions and in different sectors (women in the public sector and men in the private sector), we have chosen to show data separately for women and men and to try to illustrate the work environment and sickness absence from the partly different perspectives of women and men. Since women and men, to a large extent, work within different sectors in the labour market and in different professions, they also have different work conditions and are exposed to different risk factors. In this respect, it is also important to bear in mind that the labour market of men is more differentiated than that of women. Men are found in a broader spectrum of professions, as compared to women. The most common profession among women is assistant nurse, which occupies 15 percent of the employed women. Among men, salesman is the most common profession, occupying 4 percent of employed men (Socialstyrelsen 2009). The more limited labour market for women also has implications for their rehabilitation efforts, since they have fewer professions from which to choose.

Up until the 1980s, the sickness absence rates for women and men in Sweden were very similar (Eriksson 2009). Since then, the sickness absence rate for women has been on a higher level than for men, and in figures from 2006, the women constituted two out of three long-term sick-listed persons (Försäkringskassan 2007). Work related difficulties can be caused by shortcomings in the physical, as well as in the psycho-social, work environment. In this chapter, we concentrate on the psycho-social environment. Consequently, the main aim of the study was to explore psycho-social working conditions of importance for sickness absence. Our second aim was to find out whether there were any gender differences.

Methods

'Life and health 2008' is a postal questionnaire study regarding the health, living habits, and life conditions of the population. It was conducted during spring 2008 with a random sample of 68 710 individuals between the ages of 18 and 84 from five counties in the middle of Sweden (Värmland, Uppsala, Sörmland, Västmanland, Örebro). In total, the sample represents a population of more than one million inhabitants. The response rate was 59.2 percent. The drop-out rate was in line with what can be expected for postal surveys (Eklund, Johansson & Sundén 2002). The willingness to respond was higher for women, increased with age except for the oldest category, and increased with education level; further, the willingness to respond was higher for persons born in the Nordic countries, as compared to persons born outside the Nordic countries. Regarding occupation, it can be noted that students and unemployed persons had lower response rates. The lowest response rate was among persons who recently had immigrated to Sweden.

Since the questions analyzed in the present study were work-related, our study group is comprised of a sub sample of 19 661 (10 769 women, 8 892 men) persons of working age (18–64 years) who were employed at the time.

One oft-used method to measure psycho-social work environment, especially in relation to health, is the so called demand-control model, or job-strain model, developed by Karasek and Theorell (1990). The demand-control instrument used in this study is the Swedish version of the 11-item scale, of which 5 questions refer to the demand dimension and 6 questions, to the control dimension, which is sometimes referred to as job decision latitude. The model has also been widely used in sickness absence studies. In particular, combinations of low job control and high job demands, so called high-strain jobs, derived from the model have been associated with increased risk of sickness absence (Engström 2009). The median value for each index, consisting of the sums of the scale values, was used as the cut-off point between high and low demand and control respectively. Four job types were then constructed: low-strain jobs (low demand-high control), high-strain jobs (high demand-low control), passive jobs (low demand-low control), and active jobs (high demand-high control).

The association between job strain and the dependent variable LTSA was studied with the use of multivariate logistic regression analysis. Men and women were analyzed in separate regressions to pay special attention to possible gender differences. We also controlled for age, education, and type of employer.

Results

As shown in table 1, the most common job type, using the job-strain model, was passive, both for men and for women. Notable gender differences were that low-strain jobs were more common among men, and high-strain jobs, more common among women. The description of the population in Table 1 confirms the expected picture of the gender segregated Swedish labour market: men were typically employed by private firms, while women generally worked in the public sector. Also as expected, women were LTSA to a considerably higher extent than were men.

Table 1: Distribution of job types according to the job-strain model and background statistics.

	Men (n=8892)	Women (n=10769)
Demand Control		
Low Strain	26.8%	19.3%
Passive	38.5%	41.5%
High-Strain	19.7%	25.7%
Active	15.0%	13.6%
Age		
18–34 yrs	23.3%	26.8%
35–49 yrs	35.3%	35.8%
50–64 yrs	41.3%	37.4%
Employer		
Private employer	62.5%	31.1%
Self employed	8.8%	4.7%
Municipality	10.7%	37.3%
County	2.9%	11.3%
State	8.8%	8.4%
Other	6.3%	7.1%
Education		
Elementary school	16.3%	10.5%
High School	53.1%	49.4%
Post High School	30.6%	40.1%
Sickness Absence		
LTSA	6.4%	12.4%

The results from the multivariate logistic regressions are presented in Table 2. The odds-ratios for LTSA were studied, and special attention was given to how job strain was associated with the dependent variable. All independent variables were categorical and thus all odds ratios should be compared only to the reference categories, which all have OR=1.00 by definition in the table.

As expected, the risk for LTSA increases with age. This is true for men and women. Similar gender patterns were found for the association between education and LTSA, whereby a post-high school education seems to be protective against LTSA for both sexes. Some evidence that a public employment could be a risk factor for LTSA was suggested. Both men and women employed by the municipality had significant odds ratios higher than 1. For women, county employments, generally in the health sector, were also associated with LTSA.

Table 2: Multivariate logistic regression: Odds-Ratios (O.R) with 95% confidence intervals (C.I) for LTSA (significant ORs in bold).

	Men (n=8 892)		Women (n=10 769)	
	O.R	95% C.I	O.R	95% C.I
Demand Control				
Low Strain	1.00		1.00	
Passive	**1.27**	1.01–1.60	**1.29**	1.05–1.57
High-Strain	**1.78**	1.38–2.29	**2.45**	2.01–2.99
Active	1.07	0.78–1.45	**1.55**	1.22–1.96
Age				
18–34 yrs	1.00		1.00	
35–49 yrs	**1.57**	1.20–2.06	**1.38**	1.17–1.63
50–64 yrs	**2.38**	1.84–3.01	**1.59**	1.35–1.87
Employer				
Private employer	1.00		1.00	
Self employed	0.93	0.68–1.27	1.08	0.78–1.49
Municipality	**1.32**	1.01–1.74	**1.28**	1.10–1.49
County	0.73	0.38–1.41	**1.28**	1.03–1.59
State	1.28	0.94–1.73	1.17	0.91–1.48
Other	1.00	0.71–1.43	0.93	0.71–1.22
Education				
High School	1.00		1.00	
Elementary	1.23	0.99–1.53	0.93	0.76–1.14
Post High School	**0.54**	0.43–0.68	**0.73**	0.63–0.84

Psycho-social work environment, i.e. demand-control factors, showed strong associations with LTSA. Using low-strain jobs as the reference category, all other job types had odds ratios significantly higher than one for women. For men, this was the case for passive and high-strain jobs, but not for active jobs. High strain jobs had the highest odds ratios for both sexes. Compared to low strain jobs, the risk for LTSA was 1.8 times higher in high-strain jobs for men and almost 2.5 times higher for women. The latter was also the highest odds ratio in the entire analysis. This job type, represented through high job demands and low job control, is also the job type generally associated with ill health more generally. The main results are further highlighted in figure 1, where the four job types and their association with LTSA are illustrated.

		Low Strain jobs			Active jobs	
High		Men	Women		Men	Women
	(%)	26.8	19.3	(%)	15.0	13.6
	O.R	Ref	Ref	O.R	1.07	1.55
		Passive jobs			High Strain jobs	
Low		Men	Women		Men	Women
	(%)	38.5	41.5	(%)	19.7	25.7
	O.R	1.27	1.29	O.R	1.78	2.45
		Low			High	

Job Control (row labels); Job demands (column labels)

Figure 1: The proportion of men and women in different types of jobs according to the job-strain model and the odds-ratios (OR) for LTSA in relation to low-strain jobs.

Discussion

The study found a strong relationship between long-term sickness absence and the psycho-social work environment. Psycho-social work environment was measured through Karasek and Theorell's Demand and Control model. This is, of course, only one way to measure psycho-social work environment, but our results confirm that it is an important measure for understanding sickness absence. A social support dimension, which can act as a buffer against the negative job strain effects, is often studied as a complement to this model (Johnson & Hall 1988). In the present study, however, there were no available data to study the support dimension.

Rostila (2008) suggested that what he describes as 'healthy jobs' may be disappearing from the Swedish labour market and that the psycho-social work environment has deteriorated after the 1990s in most parts of the labour market. Our study shows a possible support for these suggestions, in that, in relation to low-strain jobs, most other job types derived from the job strain model were associated with an increased risk of LTSA. For women, this was actually true for all other job types. Rostila further considers that such results could be a sign of shortcomings of the demand-control model as a tool for analysing the complexities of the modern labour market. In our study, we still find it possible to discuss the changing labour market and its consequences on sickness absence in light of the demand-control model. Public employment, which is the most common situation for women, is partly characterized by reduced control; even someone in a managerial position is ultimately controlled by political decisions. This could provide an explanation as to why women in active jobs seem to be at higher risk for LTSA compared to women in low-strain jobs. Men in active jobs are not at higher risk for LTSA. One explanation could be that men are not employed in the public sector to nearly the same extent as women.

What has not, to our knowledge, been seen in previous studies is that even persons with passive jobs have an increased risk for LTSA. We can only speculate as to the reasons for this finding. Declining job security in terms of the increasing amount of temporary jobs and negative aspects of flexibility on the labour market is likely to be recognized also in passive jobs. One possibility is that the low-strain jobs are influenced to a lesser extent by this development in the labour market and are thus still 'healthy jobs'. Perhaps an even more likely explanation for the association between passive jobs and LTSA can be found in the increasing inequalities in society. People employed in passive jobs are likely to be increasingly vulnerable to subordination in working life and to social inequalities. Wilkinson & Picket (2009) claim that social inequality is the foundation for ill-health and other social problems.

The much higher odds ratios for women working in high strain jobs, as compared to men with similar working conditions, also requires discussion. One possible explanation is the combined impact of domestic responsibilities and job strain, so-called double exposure. Swedish women carry out about two thirds of all unpaid work related to the home (Krantz & Östergren 2001). In the case of a woman working in a high strain job, this double exposure could have an added impact on health and, by extension, sickness absence.

As in all cross-sectional studies, causal relationships cannot be studied. Only associations between variables are possible to detect.

References

Eklund, Maria, Birgitta Johansson & Annika Sundén 2002. *Sjukskrivnas syn på hälsa och arbete* (Sickness absentees' view on health and work. In Swedish). Stockholm, Swedish Social Insurance Agency

Engström, Lars-Gunnar 2009. *Sickness Absence in Sweden. Its relation to Work, Health and Social Insurance Factors.* Diss. Karlstad University, Karlstad

Eriksson, Ulla-Britt 2009. *Man är ju inte mer än människa – Långtidssjukskrivning ur ett emotionellt, relationellt och strukturellt perspektiv.* Diss. Karlstad University, Karlstad

Esping-Andersen, Gösta 1990. *Three worlds of welfare capitalism.* Cambridge, Polity Press

Försäkringskassan 2007. *Långtidssjukskrivna – demografi, arbete, yrke, diagnos, sjukpenningrätt och återgång till arbete 2003, 2005 och 2006.* Stockholm, Social Insurance Agency

Johnson, J.V. & E.M. Hall 1988. 'Job Strain, Work Place Social Support, and Cardiovascular Disease: A Cross-Sectional Study of a Random Sample of the Swedish Working Population'. *American Journal of Public Health*, 78, 1336–1342

Karasek, Robert & Töres Theorell 1990. *Healthy Work: Stress, Productivity, and the Reconstruction of Working Life.* New York, Basic Books

Krantz, Gunilla & Per-Olof Östergren 2001. 'Double exposure. The combined impact of domestic responsibilities and job strain on common symptoms in employed Swedish women'. *European Journal of Public Health*, 11, 413–419

Rostila, Mikael 2008. 'The Swedish labour market in the 1990s: The very last of the healthy jobs?' *Scandinavian Journal of Public Health*, 36:126–134

Socialdepartementet 2008. *En förnyad folkhälsopolitik.* Prop 2007/08:110. Stockholm, Socialdepartementet

Socialstyrelsen 2009. *Folkhälsorapport 2009.* Stockholm, Socialstyrelsen

Wilkinson, Richard & Kate Picket 2009. *The Spirit Level: Why More Equal Societies Almost Always Do Better.* Bloomsbury Publishing Plc

Chapter 11

Working part-time for the sake of health

Lena Ede

Summary

The Swedish labour market is gender segregated both by different sectors (men in the private sector and women mainly in the public sector) and by working hours. It is more common for men to work full-time and for women to work part-time. For women working in municipal elderly care, part-time work is even more frequent than full-time work. Working part-time in a low-paying job usually results in economic difficulties. The most common reason for working part-time is the lack of full-time jobs, but it is also possible to decline an offer to work full-time for other reasons. Taking care of one's children is one and taking care of one's health is another. This chapter explores the relation between part-time work and care workers' health, in particular, how part-time work can be understood as a necessary personal strategy for avoiding long-term sickness absence. The chapter is based on data from five different studies of municipality elderly care, where organisational models aiming to increase the number of full-time jobs for care workers were implemented. The care workers revealed a picture of physically and psychosocially demanding work. Despite the need for a full-time salary, many of them continued to work part-time as a strategy for avoiding various health problems and sickness absence.

Introduction

The focus in this chapter is on care workers (including assistant nurses) in municipal elderly care and their working conditions. They represent the largest professional group on the labour market in Sweden. They work on the frontline and provide care and help to people who need assistance in their everyday life; of this group, 87 per cent are women (Statistiska Centralbyrån 2009). For these women, part-time work is the most frequent form of employment. The most common reason for working part-time is the lack of full-time jobs, with illness or inability to cope with working conditions coming in second, followed by care for children/adults (Larsson 2009). Throughout this chapter, I will focus on the relation between part-time work and care workers' health, but I will first say something about part-time work and part-time unemployment in general.

In Sweden, the normal work week is set at 40 hours per week (SOU 2002). This does not necessarily mean that all vocational groups work the same number of hours. For many shift-workers, full-time is 30–35 hours per week (Larsson 2009). For care workers, a full-time position is generally 37 hours per week. The most frequent level of working time for the care workers is between 75 and 80 percent of full-time employment.

Working part-time may be voluntary as the result of an active choice to suit an individual's life circumstances, if his or her financial situation makes this possible. Working part-time may be involuntary, if the employer does not offer full-time employment, or if the working conditions are too demanding to cope with. Working part-time may also be a temporary choice for parents who want to reduce their full-time position by up to 25 per cent until their children reach the age of eight. The differences between these various forms of part-time work should be taken into account, since the latter is based on a full-time position, which provides the possibility of returning to full-time at any point. Thus, voluntary part-time work is worth maintaining, but it is of considerable importance to come to terms with involuntary part-time work, since this entails part-time unemployment.

Part-time unemployment usually results in various types of financial problems, such as difficulty in supporting oneself both in the current situation and after retirement. Additionally, working part-time influences health insurance, parental insurance, and unemployment benefits. Since June 2008, a reduction in the unemployment insurance for the part-time unemployed has been carried out by the Swedish government. The number of days of compensation has been reduced from 300 to 75. No changes have been made for the full-time unemployed.

Before 2005, public statistics on part-time work (and thus part-time unemployment) were unavailable, and this makes it difficult to measure the extent of part-time work over time. Another measurement problem arises from the fact that there is no established definition of part-time unemployment (Forsell & Jonsson 2005). In public statistics, the term used is 'underemployed', which refers to individuals who are involuntarily working fewer hours than they would like to. In the first quarter of 2009, 319 000 people were underemployed in Sweden; 131 000 men and 187 000 women (Statistiska Centralbyrån 2009).

Part-time work and part-time unemployment are most widespread among women, primarily among women working in low-paying jobs, like those in the care sector. It is also women in the public sector, particularly those working in the health and care professions, who show the highest increase in long-term sickness absence (SOU 2005). In this group, there is a large number of part-time sickness absence and early retirement (Hartman & Jönsson 2008). The highest level is found among care workers aged 55 or older (SKL 2008). One reason for this is that the demand for increased productivity, together with continual reorganisations, affects the psychosocial work environment. The pace and demands have increased to such an extent that part-time work is regarded as a necessary solution in order to cope with daily work (SOU 2005).

It has been shown that work-related problems such as pain, tiredness and exhaustion are more frequent among care workers in elderly care, as compared to workers in other professions (Trygdegård 2005). A survey of research on Nordic elderly care revealed that the workload has increased during the last years. The work is more demanding, both physically and mentally, and there is a high incidence of work-related illness and injuries (Szebehely 2005; Hammarström & Hensing 2008).

The study

I have studied the implementation of new ways to increase the number of full-time jobs for care workers in municipal elderly care. In the organisations I analysed, the working schedule had been recently rearranged. This was understood as essential to keeping within the budgets. My aim was to study the consequences of relating to the new way of organising the working hours for the care workers in their every day life. I was also interested in understanding the care workers' beliefs and preferences about choosing to work full-time or not.

The data were collected during 2000–2005 in the form of qualitative interviews in five different municipalities. I interviewed approximately 165 care workers in their working environment during their working hours. Some of them were interviewed together in groups, others, in one-to-one conversation. The organisation of the interviews depended substantially on the respondents' working conditions and how much time they could spend with me. I selected teams from different parts of the elderly care facility in order to get as many different opinions as possible. The results have been reported to each municipality (Ede & Sjödén 2002; Ede & Karlsson 2003; Ede 2005a, 2005b; Ede & Strandell 2005). When working on the present discussion, I analyzed the data a second time. I have focused on the relation between part-time work and care workers' health, and, in particular, how part-time work is understood as a necessary means of avoiding long-term sickness absence.

Considerations regarding the choice of working hours

The new organization of working hours made it possible to work full-time. Nevertheless, quite a few care workers declined the opportunity and continued to work part-time. The most common reason cited was consideration for their children. This is not surprising. There are many studies supporting these findings (e.g. Bekkengen 2002). The difficulty to combine full-time work with parenthood was emphasized by Thomsson (1998) more than a decade ago. The care workers who had small children and the financial means chose to continue working part-time.

My results also show that the need to help aged parents affects the choice of working hours. 'I can't work full-time now that my parents are old and need a lot of help' was a typical comment. Research in Sweden on caring for relatives is limited, but Ulmanen (2009) shows that middle-aged women who provide help to relatives every day or several times a week prefer to work part-time.

I will not here discuss in detail family care and the possible preferences underlying choices of working hours. I will instead concentrate on the second most common reason for working part-time, namely, to avoid illness, health problems, and sickness absence, which may result from the heavy work load. One care worker expressed it in the following terms: 'Being able to work full-time is good, but I don't know whether I can manage to work full-time with such a tough job'. She was positive about the opportunity of working full-time, but she doubted whether she could cope with it throughout her working life in light of her own health. The opportunity to influence one's hours of work was seen as a gain by the majority, still many of the workers did not want to work full-time for personal reasons.

In answer to my question regarding the choice of working hours, a group of care workers said, 'None of us have gone over to full-time. It is too demanding, and we can't cope'. Their opinions were based upon many years of care work. Another care worker, who had experienced almost a whole working life in the care sector, explained the motivation for her choice as follows: 'I have worked for 40 years with demanding care work and have aches and pains. Now I really need to work full-time as the salary is low – but I can't manage it, it's too demanding'. In her case, the money was less important than her health.

Others described their own ambivalence about balancing the desire to increase their salary with the risk of not being able to cope with full-time work. The perverse choice of more money at the cost of one's health was expressed by a care worker in the following manner: 'Offering full-time employment without altering the work environment is like putting a bowl of sweets in front of a diabetic'. This finding is supported by Båvner (2001) who, in his doctoral thesis, showed that women with physically demanding jobs worked part-time to a greater extent than women with less physically demanding jobs. Apart from this, there is little research indicating health as a reason for choosing to work part-time.

What did the care workers mean when they said the work was demanding? In my data, I found expressions describing the work as physically demanding.

Lifting and moving elderly people, washing their clothes, and cleaning their homes, as well as travelling between the homes of different care recipients, cause physical wear and tear. For instance, the pressure on the lumbar region for an individual bent over another person to help them get out of bed is equivalent to carrying an object weighing 200 kilograms (Kommunal 2005).

I also found expressions describing the psychosocial aspects of the work, regarding preparation for the unexpected, relationships and emotions, and bad conscience when the ideal of good care had to take a back seat. This psychosocial aspect of the work is more difficult to measure, but it is no less demanding than the physical. Time for reflection is probably just as important as the time for rest after having completed a demanding physical task. This mixture of physical and psychosocial work seems to be crucial when the care workers describe their work as demanding. One of them summarised the complexity of the work in the following terms:

> A certain basic physical fitness is necessary. Your body suffers wear and tear. There is a lot of lifting and carrying. And a lot of responsibility. We are the first to visit a person if something has happened. And then there is a lot of cleaning and other stuff. I am responsible for the vehicles, and now we have to get the winter tyres on. Then there are all the purchases.

This combination of duties – the demanding physical tasks together with the responsibility for another person's wellbeing – is one of the reasons why the work is experienced as demanding.

Being prepared for the unexpected

Even though the care workers describe their working day as governed by timetables and routines, it is filled with the unexpected as well. The strain of being attentive to the needs of another and being prepared for the unexpected, is described by a care worker working in a home for dementia patients:

> You must be attentive at all times. You cannot relax even when you have a break, and when you've gone on like this for a long time, you get tired. It is a continual state of emergency and it's chaotic and sometimes you have to answer the same question thirty times. It's mentally very trying.

Dementia involves a disturbed memory function and unpredictable mood swings, conditions which were well known to the care workers and accepted as a part of the disease. One group working in a home for those diagnosed with dementia recounted how they had to apply a large measure of flexibility to keep the care recipients in a good mood, so that they got on well together and avoid being pinched, which could occur very unexpectedly. This produced a tiredness described by one of care workers in the following way: 'It feels as though your head is crawling with ants when you go home from work'. Another one explained that 'it can take several hours or even a day before your head is clear again'. These elusive aspects and experiences were perceived as very demanding among the care workers.

Wångblad (2009) found similar results in her study of dementia care. What the care workers experienced as demanding was not merely the physical aspects of the work but also the misunderstandings and communication problems, which arose when they were about to lift, support and move the care recipients. It was difficult to understand whether the care recipient would cope with the same situation from one day to the next, since the symptoms of the illness varied substantially. This uncertainty made moving and lifting the care recipients especially demanding (Wångblad 2009). Being prepared for the unexpected is one aspect of the invisible work going on in the mind, and this seems to be a fundamental reason why the work is experienced as difficult to handle.

Relationships and emotions

The care workers have to deal with feelings on a daily basis in the sense that they are faced with the care recipients' expressions of emotion. This emotional work seems to be a key factor when care workers attempt to explain what they mean when they report that their work is demanding. For a type of work to be considered emotional work in Hochschild's (1983) sense, it has to involve three ingredients. First, there must be face-to-face or voice-to-voice contact. Second, the employee must generate an emotional state in the other person (for instance, a sense of security), and third, the employer must control the expression of emotion through training or supervision. The care workers provided many examples of the first two and even some of the third as well. In two of the municipalities, the care workers received training in common values.

A care worker explained the emotional work in the following way:

> We have a tough job, but that's true of everybody working with people. There might be a day when you don't feel in good shape, but you can't show it. You have to be nice and kind, don't you… as long as you're dealing with people. If you're working with a machine, it doesn't matter so much. You can kick it if you want, but you can't kick the legs of one of the old people I work with. We have to accept a lot, but we can't pay them back. That places a greater strain on you. Physically it is, of course, demanding but it's worse mentally.

The care worker reveals an understanding of challenges confronting other professions working in close relationship with other people, but she emphasises that she faces people in the final stages of their life. Providing care for very old people entails having death as a constant companion, and several respondents described the difficulty of defending themselves against emotional reactions. One care worker who worked in a home for people diagnosed with dementia expressed it in the following way: 'Our care recipients come here and stay until they die. You form attachments to many of them. It's obvious you're affected when somebody dies'. Working in elderly care, in itself, entails taking care of old people during the last years of their life, and awareness of this was self-evident among the care workers. Another said, 'Even though you do as much as you can for them, they won't get better … in the end they die and this is obviously hard'. Coping with one's own feelings is an aspect of the psychosocially demanding nature of the work.

Coping with others' feelings is another aspect. The emotion work the care workers describe requires a lot of energy in the sense that one must face the care recipients' mood swings, without revealing what one really feels. The care workers often dwelt on the fact that there was a difference between working with people and with things and that suppressing one's own feelings to remain outwardly friendly placed them under a mental strain. They reported receiving both scoldings and blows from care recipients, even though they did their best to understand the latters' illnesses.

Emotion work, according to Hochschild (1983) is based on relationships, in this case between care workers and care recipients. It is carried out by the care worker in a demanding work process. Suppressing the spontaneous feelings that arise and then finding a more appropriate feeling to be shown is an expression of this work. One can either pretend to have the correct feelings – what Hochschild terms surface action – or one can actually generate the feeling that one is supposed to feel – so-called deep action. This must bee done without revealing feelings of tiredness so that the work seems effortless. It is hard to maintain a distinction between what one really feels and what one shows. Hochschild (1983) describes this state as one of emotive dissonance.

The care workers gave expression to the feeling of guilt by speaking of their own sense of inadequacy. One care worker described it as follows: 'I had a bad conscience when I got home. I knew that I hadn't done a good job. I hadn't done what I should have'. She carried out the tasks she had been given, but this was not sufficient for her to feel satisfied. There was something lacking. She gave expression to her sense of powerlessness thus:

> But what sort of quality is that. These are people. You can't just come and put on a stocking and then leave. Then you would be a machine. And on many occasions they have something which worries them or they are sad about. And want to talk. If you just stand there restless and wanting to leave, they notice. They really want to talk about things and you can't just stand there washing up or turn your back on them and make a noise. And they might not hear very well … and I keep an eye on the clock all the time. It doesn't feel right.

For her, an essential part of providing good care is fostering a relationship, which is precisely what she did not have time to do, and this led her to feel dissatisfied with her own work.

To know how each care recipient wanted the task done seemed to be a precondition for providing good quality in the physical tasks. As one of the care workers expressed it: 'It's not enough to do what you're supposed to. You also have to learn how to act towards each care recipient and to do it as they want it done'. When the care workers described their work as 'well done', they meant that they not only completed the task but that they also did so in 'the right way', that is, in the way the care recipient wanted it. Knowledge about how the care recipient wanted it was grounded in established relationships with the care recipients. Building relationships in order to learn 'how they like their pudding', as one of them put it, was seen to be an essential aspect of doing a good job. Having the ambition to deal with the care recipients on the basis of their personalities, with their differing needs, values and attitudes, means that there are many relationships to take into account. One care worker explained it thus:

> You go from a dementia sufferer to one who is physical ill and to one who is dying. You have to adapt in so many different ways. And in my mind I am already on my way to the next care recipient. Home-help care workers have to meet all those over 65 who are living at home and receive the home-help service. They can have all kinds of diagnoses. You really learn to adjust to each person you're with. The way you behave with Olga is not the same as with Kalle. You have to adapt to each. And you don't have time. There's always a rush to do the cleaning and washing. It's in the car that you adapt.

In answer to my question about how she felt after a day's work, she replied: 'Yes, it's tough. Especially when I work until four. Then I'm exhausted'. According to Hochschild (1983), anyone who is expected to conduct personal encounters in a work environment that does not provide proper opportunities to establish relationships due to lack of time risks ill-health. Hochschild maintains that those who are too involved in their professional role risk burnout and those who distance themselves risk either having a guilty conscience or distancing themselves from the feelings of guilt and becoming cynical. In the quotation above, the care worker said she 'had to adapt in the car' and that 'in her mind she was on her way to the next care recipient'. This indicates that the time between completing one encounter and preparing for the next is too short. As Hochschild sees it, this means risking illness.

The ideal of good care vs. the reality

The conflict between the ideal and norms for good care and the work that was possible to perform seemed to lead to frustration among the care workers. This was especially apparent when they were forced to hold back their own values in order to carry out the work within the limits laid down by their employers. 'I don't want my old parents to be treated like this', said one care worker when describing her work. The organisation of work did not allow her to provide the type of care that she wanted to in order to feel that she had done a good job. The inability to feel pride in one's work may be a contributory reason that the job is perceived as demanding.

The care workers described how the work had changed through reorganisation, economy measures, narrower time limits, and increased administrative responsibility. One of the work teams reported that the financial situation came up at every staff meeting. This was unwelcome, they claimed, since they considered it to be a management issue, and not something to be discussed with the staff. Information about economic considerations and demanding budgets created anxiety. The main concern was whether they would still have a job if there were staff reductions. One care worker put it like this:

> If you've worked in care for a number of years and continually hear that you have to save and save. Never anything that is positive. You get tired of hearing it. You save and niggle over the timetable and scrape and save. That's what it's been like as long as I've been here. It's hard continually living with this worry.

Another consequence of reorganisation was that there were new tasks for the care workers, involving documentation and paperwork, i.e. staffing and making timetables. These tasks were conceived of as managerial ones that took time from what they called 'real work', taking care of people. This type of peripheral work (Semmer 2010) created work stress that one of the care workers described in the following manner:

> You have to do so many new things which are not part of the job. All this paperwork. Can't we spend the time on those who live here instead? Sometimes it feels like… shall I help the person who needs me or write down what I have almost forgotten.

Not having enough time to carry out one's duties in a manner that corresponds to the norms for good care seemed to cause major practical and personal problems. This causes a moral conflict which, according to Stone (2000), can lead to ill health. Inherent in care giving, according to Szebehely (2005), is a limitlessness; it is difficult for the individual to know when sufficient care has been provided. A consequence of this limitlessness is a general sense of inadequacy. In a study by Gustafsson & Szebehely (2005), the feeling of inadequacy emerged as a particularly serious and growing work-environment problem. In my study, one of the care workers summarized this sense of inadequacy in the following way:

> With the diminishing resources you have, all you concentrate on is ensuring that the care recipients don't notice. Then it's you who suffers. You feel you don't really have time. You work as much as you can and still feel you're inadequate.

Conclusion

The aim of this chapter has been to understand the relation between part-time work and care workers' health, and in particular how part-time work is understood as a necessary strategy for avoiding long-term sickness absence. I have explored two crucial questions. First, how voluntary is the choice of part-time work? Second, how are part-time work practices related to care workers' preferences and ideas about their own mental and physical health?

My findings show that the fundamental problem occurs when care workers need to work full-time for economical reasons but find that they cannot cope because of the psychically and psychosocially demanding work tasks. For many, the choice of working part-time for the sake of one's own health becomes the best solution, but not an ideal one. Furthermore, part-time work does not correspond with many of the care workers' own fundamental wishes and interests.

From the descriptions the care workers gave in my interviews, there emerges an overall picture of physically demanding work combined with considerable psychosocial demands. When they described their work as demanding, they were referring to many kinds of 'wear and tear'. Their work was often done under time pressure and emotional strain. They talked about being prepared for the unexpected as one aspect of the invisible psychosocial work. They also had to cope with emotions, both the care recipients' and their own.

The care workers talked about the moral conflict between their own ideals of good care and what was possible within the limits laid down by their employer. They also talked about time-consuming paper work and feelings of inadequateness. The mixture of the physical and psychosocial work seems to be crucial for understanding why so many care workers go on working part-time even when they get the opportunity to work full-time. For them, this is a strategy for avoiding health problems that lead to sickness absence.

References

Bekkengen, Lisbeth 2002. *Man får välja – Om föräldraskap och föräldraledighet i arbetsliv och familjeliv.* Malmö, Liber Ekonomi

Båvner, Per 2001. *Half full or Half empty? Part time work and well-being among Swedish women.* Stockholm, Stockholms universitet

Ede, Lena & Lisbet Sjödén 2002. *Högre sysselsättningsgrad – ett sätt att göra vård- och omsorgsarbetet mera attraktivt?* IKU-rapport 2002:1. Karlstad, Karlstads universitet

Ede, Lena & Lena Karlsson 2003. *Resurs- och bemanningsteam – en arbetstidsmodell. Utvärdering av ett projekt i Årjängs kommun.* IKU-rapport 2003:2. Karlstad, Karlstads universitet

Ede, Lena 2005a. *Äldreomsorgens organisering. Utvärdering av projekt Tänk Vidare i Hammarö kommun.* IKU-rapport 2005:5. Karlstad, Karlstads universitet

Ede, Lena 2005b. *Heltid åt alla – Filosofi i vården. Utvärdering av ett förändringsarbete inom äldreomsorgen i Torsby kommun.* IKU-rapport 2005:8. Karlstad, Karlstads universitet

Ede, Lena & Barbro Strandell 2005. *En Hel Del – Munkforsmodellen. Utvärdering av ett förändringsarbete inom äldre- och handikappomsorgen i Munkfors kommun.* IKU-rapport 2005:9. Karlstad, Karlstads universitet

Forsell, Johanna & Inger Johansson 2005. *Deltidsarbetslöshet och deltidsarbete i Europa, Förklaringsmodeller och statistik.* Workingpaper från HELA-projektet 2005:6. Stockholm, Arbetslivsinstitutet

Gunnarsson, Evy & Marta Szebehely eds. 2009. *Genus i omsorgens vardag.* Stockholm, Gothia Förlag

Gustafsson, Rolf Å. & Martha Szebehely 2005. *Arbetsvillkor och styrning i äldreomsorgens hierarki – en enkätstudie bland personal och politiker.* Rapport i socialt arbete no. 114–2005. Stockholm, Stockholms universitet, Institutionen för socialt arbete, Socialhögskolan

Hammarström, Anne & Gunnel Hensing 2008. *Folkhälsofrågor ur ett genusperspektiv. Arbetsmarknad, maskuliniteter, medikalisering och könsrelaterad våld.* Östersund, Statens Folkhälsoinstitut

Hartman, Laura & Lisa, Jönsson 2008. 'Deltidsarbete och deltidsförmåner i Sverige'. Hartman, Laura ed. *Välfärd på deltid,* Stockholm, SNS Förlag, 21–62

Hochschild, Arlie Russell 1983. *The managed heart – Commerzialisation of Human Feeling.* Berkely, University of California Press

Larsson, Mats 2009. *Arbetstider år 2009. Heltids- och deltidsarbete, vanligen arbetad tid och arbetstidens förläggning efter klass och kön år 1990–2009.* Stockholm, LO Faktamaterial/statistik, Arbetslivsenheten

Kommunal 2005. *Sexton år av smärta och besvär. En rapport om kommunalarnas arbetsmiljö och hälsa år 1988–2003.* Stockholm, Svenska Kommunalarbetarförbundet

Statistiska Centralbyrån 2009. *Arbetsmarknadssituationen för hela befolkningen 15–74 år, AKU 4:e kvartalet 2009. Tema – Undersysselsatta.* www.scb.se/Pages/PressRelease_288162.aspx

Semmer, Norbert et al. 2010. 'Illegitime Tasks and Counterproductive Work Behaviour.' *Applied Psychology* 2010, 59 (1), 70–76

SOU 2002. *Arbetstiden – livets gränser. 2002:49.* Stockholm, Fritzes

SOU 2005 *Makt att forma samhället och sitt eget liv – jämställdhetspolitiken mot nya mål, 2005:66.* Stockholm, Fritzes

Stone, Deborah 2000. 'Caring by the book'. Harrington Meyer M. ed.: *Care Work, Gender, labour and the welfare state.* New York, Routhledge

Szebehely, Marta 2005. 'Äldreomsorgen i Norden – verksamhet, forskning och statistik'. Szhebehely, Marta ed.: *Äldreomsorgsforskning i Norden. En kunskapsöversikt,* 21–49

Szhebehely, Marta ed. 2005. *Äldreomsorgsforskning i Norden. En kunskapsöversikt.* Köpenhamn. Nordiska ministerrådet

Thomsson, Helene 1998. *Anpasningens pris: Kvinnors liv i vård och vardag.* Stockholm, Förlagshuset Gothia

Trygdegård, Gun-Britt 2005. 'Äldreomsorgspersonalens arbetsvillkor i Norden – en forskningsöversikt.' Szebehely, Marta ed.: *Äldreomsorgsforskning i Norden. En kunskapsöversikt,* 143–163

Ulmanen, Petra 2009. 'Anhörigomsorgens pris för döttrar och söner till omsorgsbehövande äldre'. Gunnarsson, Evy & Marta Szebehely eds.: *Genus i omsorgens vardag,* 117–131

Wångblad Cristina 2009. 'Experiences of physical strain during person transfer situations in dementia care units'. *Scandinavian Journal of Caring Sciences.* Published on line: 19 Aug 2009

Chapter 12

The benefits of nature and culture activities on health, environment and wellbeing: A presentation of three evaluation studies among persons with chronic illnesses and sickness absence in Norway

Kari Batt-Rawden & Gunnar Tellnes

Summary

Researchers have investigated the potential of nature-culture-health activities in terms of their health-promoting properties. The aim of this chapter is to present results from three evaluation studies focusing on how art, music, nature and culture have a beneficial impact on health and wellbeing. The first evaluation study describes the subjective experiences of people partaking in nature-culture-health activities at the National Centre for Nature-Culture-Health (NaCuHeal) in Asker, a municipality west of Oslo. The second evaluation study highlights the way that music can act as a sort of folk-medical practice in our contemporary culture to maintain, improve, or change health status, though it is administered in a non-professional setting. The third evaluation paper presents results from a study conducted by Eastern Norway Research Institute [ENRI] in collaboration with the Fron Rehabilitation Centre, Norway in 2008–2009. A common theme, and hence a major finding, is that nature-culture-health experiences may, from a salutogenic perspective, help participants to construct a meaning, to identify coping mechanisms, and to revitalize the energetic and resourceful parts of the self. This kind of research could stimulate future health promotion and interdisciplinary cooperation in rehabilitation programs.

Introduction

This chapter present results from three evaluation studies focusing on how art, music, and nature-culture-health activities may have a beneficial impact on health and wellbeing. In recent years, some researchers have investigated the potential of nature and cultural activities in terms of their health-promoting properties (Tellnes 1996; 2003a; 2009; Konlaan 2001; Konlaan, Bygren & Johansson 2000; Karaberg, Tellnes & Karaberg 2004; Batt-Rawden & Tellnes 2005; Batt-Rawden 2010; 2010a; Batt-Rawden & Tellnes 2010). This research has opened up a range of new and important questions that warrant empirical investigation. We still need to know more about the practices and processes by which engagement with nature and culture may function in life-enhancing and health-promoting ways as well as in relation to sickness absence and rehabilitation (see also chapter 5). It is not enough, in other words, to discover correlations between cultural activities and wellbeing; it is much more interesting to understand how such activities come to be associated with wellbeing – and to understand the practices that lead to this outcome.

In wealthy countries, illness has been shown to be linked primarily to social and lifestyle-related factors lying outside the reach of traditional health-care systems (Tellnes 1990; see also chapter 5). Changes in health and sickness[1], long term absence from work, and disability pension have increased over the last few years, and these are often an indication of a failure to cope despite apparent good health (Alexanderson 2005). The sickness-panorama of today

---

[1] Sickness is defined as the sick role some people assume when they have a disease or an illness. Sickness is a state of social dysfunction. A person receiving a sickness certificate may assume a sick role by being absent from work. However, some people may assume no sick role, for example, those who continue their work as usual without receiving a sickness certificate, even when they have a disease or illness (Tellnes 1990).

has changed significantly in relation to the possibilities that modern medicine offers. Muscle and joint-pains, depressions and drug-abuse will demand among professionals and politicians to think outside the frame. Insecurity and intensity in the work life is problematic to many. The time-trap is pressuring families with little children. They can't cope, despite good intentions about an inclusive work-life (Holmboe-Ottesen & Tellnes 2005, 22).

Illness, disease, and sickness have a major impact on the economic situation and on the wellbeing of an individual in any society. Tomorrow's society will most probably focus more on what strengthens health, namely the salutogenic,[2] or health-causing, factors (Tellnes 2009). The medicalisation of unpleasant or stressful aspects of daily life may only add to an already large amount of over-treatment and to the growth of health-care costs (Williams, Gabe & Calnan 2000). In Norway, for example, about 50% of those who receive disability pension have been diagnosed with muscular diseases, closely followed by those diagnosed with psychosocial problems, i.e. anxiety and depression (NOU White Paper 1998). From this perspective, health is a metaphor rich in its power to signify a range of meanings, from the narrowly technical to the all-embracing moral or philosophical (Gerhardt 2000; Crawford 2000; Williams, Gabe & Calnan 2000; Naidoo & Wills 2000). Health, in this sociological conceptualization, is not a pre-given or immutable state, but socially and actively produced, performed, or negotiated as a feature of ordinary people in their everyday lives.

The illness experience

The subjective dimension provides, as it were, a mediator of health strategies and coping mechanisms at both the individual and the group level. Debates centering on this theme have emphasized social and personal resources, in addition to physical capacities. Recent research shows how working conditions and burdens in private life seem to have an impact on the development of illness and sickness absence, reinforcing the perception of the situation as involving a total life burden. From this viewpoint, the performance of health-promoting

---

[2] A salutogenic perspective emphasizes factors contributing to health and wellbeing and those that predicts a good outcome (Antonovsky 1987; Suominen & Lindström 2008).

activities involves an element of participation and empowerment (Aldridge 1996). The sociology of illness experience should be attentive to people's everyday lives, how they live in spite of illness, and what type of strategies they use to simply 'get by' in their lives (Conrad 1987). From this perspective, the subjective reality of the sufferer needs to be taken into account in health research by exploring the relationships between individuals, crisis, and sickness, for example, by focusing on 'concepts such as stress, 'sense of coherence', insecurity and lack of control' (Blaxter 2000, 34). An 'outsider' perspective, i.e. that of health professionals, often minimizes or ignores the subjective experience of illness itself (Conrad 1987). According to Radley (1997), the strategies people use to deal with illness and disease are 'all important features to be examined'. Recent research shows how working conditions and burdens in private life seem to have an impact on the development of illness and sickness absence, reinforcing the perception of a total life burden situation (Rønning, Batt-Rawden & Solheim 2008; see also chapter 13). Health is not a pre-given or immutable state, but socially and actively produced, performed, or negotiated as a feature of ordinary people in their everyday lives. This process becomes most apparent when doctors and their patients disagree about the significance or meaning of symptoms and interpretation of illnesses or disease.

Challenges for health promotion and public health

The experience of chronic and life-threatening illness is often accompanied by circumstances that lead to the loss of self (Charmaz 1991). This loss is often accompanied by aesthetic deprivation which exacerbates the problem (Goffman 1961). Maintaining one's identity and cultivating strategies of self-care in everyday life are thus a vital part of the project of improving public health. This means that health promotion requires the full participation of the people concerned and cannot afford to ignore lived experiences, personal resources, and strategies for coping with adverse circumstances or life complications (Charmaz 1999). The World Health Organization (WHO) has been responsible for stimulating the debate about definitions of health, focusing on how individuals or groups are able to realise aspirations and satisfy needs and how people may change or cope with their environment. The shaping of health-promoting settings at work, in hospitals, in schools, and in local communities has therefore been significantly supported by the WHO (Tellnes

2009). To be able to meet these new challenges for health promotion and public health, new methods and approaches involving interdisciplinary collaborations and cooperation need to be developed and tested. In relation to these themes, it is important to document scientifically how and why participation in nature-culture-health activities may prove beneficial for individuals with long term illnesses.

Aims of this chapter

The overall aim of this chapter is to show how art, music, and nature-culture-health activities may have beneficial impact on sickness absence, health, wellbeing, and rehabilitation. Three evaluation studies will then be presented, which have main aims in common (Batt-Rawden & Tellnes 2005; Batt-Rawden & Tellnes 2005a; Batt-Rawden & Tellnes 2010). Each study will be presented with its specific aims, methods, and results. Major results, similarities, connections, and patterns from all three studies will be brought together at the end. The reason behind this presentation is to find common ground in order to begin to build a scientific platform to show the effect of nature and culture activities on health.

Evaluation study 1: Nature-Culture-Health Activities (NaCuHeal)

The first evaluation study (Batt-Rawden & Tellnes 2005) describes the subjective experiences of people partaking in Nature-Culture-Health activities at the National Centre for Nature-Culture-Health (NaCuHeal) in Asker, a municipality west of Oslo. The purpose of the NaCuHeal Centre is to promote health, good environment, and quality of life, and there have since 1994 been several experiments, in which people on long-term sick leave, in rehabilitation or on social support have been helped to find their own talents and capacities in order to maintain function and pleasure in work. The physicians, psychiatrists, or health professionals often refer people long-term certified as sick to the centre, though participation is fully voluntary. Some people take their own initiative or are recommended by friends to contact the centre. The most typical diagnoses are muscular diseases, closely followed by psychosocial problems, i.e. anxiety, depression, chronic fatigue, or stress-symptoms from a severe burn-out. In general, diagnoses, illnesses, and diseases are not a recurrent theme in discussions, and these are only introduced as a theme if participants themselves initiate such topics. At the Nature-Culture-Health Centre, what is desirable is the participation and positive interactions among persons of all ages, health status, philosophies, and social positions. The idea is that such a meeting place between practitioners and theorists, and between the presently well and the presently not so well, will be stimulating and enlightening to most. Through participation in Nature-Culture-Health groups, the individual are given the opportunity to bring his or her own ideas to life and to focus on positive and creative activities outside oneself. Persons with different health problems may forget their health-related and social problems for a while. The NaCuHeal activities may nourish other aspects of one's personality that may also need development, attention, and strengthening in order to prepare for community and new social networks (Tellnes 2003). The concept of Nature-Culture-Health is based on the idea of stimulating to wholeness thinking and creativity within the Nature-Culture-Health interplay (Tellnes 1996; Karaberg, Tellnes& Karabeg 2004). This is done by emphasizing:

- Nature, out-door life, and environmental activities.
- Culture, art, physical activity, and sustainable food.
- Health promotion, prevention, therapy, and rehabilitation.

The intention is to:
- Increase participant's own empowerment and participation in activities in relation to strengthening their own health, quality of life, and function.
- Create a growth in social networks that are encouraging and stimulating.
- Motivate participants to increase their ability to work and to explore ways of coping with day-to-day activities.

According to the purpose of the NaCuHeal Centre, every individual will experience different group activities that show how dance, music, physical activity, painting, nature walks, hiking, gardening, and contact with pets can have a positive though indirect effect on their zest for life, inspiration, and desire for rehabilitation. The participants can choose for themselves which activities they want to engage in, and individuals do sometimes participate in several activities during a week, for example, painting, nature walks, and choir practice. There are usually about twelve ongoing health-promoting group activities each week, and each are scheduled for about two hours. The activity groups are led by professionals, e.g. musicians, artists, teachers, or health workers, and some group leaders were recruited from among those participating in one or several groups for a longer period of time. The NaCuHeal Centre has about 400 people participating in different activities during one week. For persons long-term certified sick for more than eight weeks, this may be a method for rehabilitation and return to work (Tellnes 1996; Pauswang 1999).

There were two aims of the first evaluation study (1)

1. To evaluate health, quality of life, and function among participants in Nature-Culture-Health activities in the local community.
2. To investigate if, how, and why participation in such activities affects people's own subjective perceptions of health and wellbeing.

Evaluation methodology

The Nature-Culture-Health Centre (NaCuHeal) in Asker in the county of Akershus, in collaboration with Akershus University College in Southern Norway, conducted a qualitative evaluation study in 2002, analysing benefits to the health and wellbeing of participants in different group activities. A total of 30 men and 16 women aged 30–79 years old participated voluntarily and were interviewed for about an hour each using a semi-structured interview guide. All informants were analysed according to group attendance, duration, regularity, and social background, subjective opinions, and beliefs. Patterns, tendencies, and main characteristics have been explored, and the main results are presented through typical quotations from the informants, along with the quantification of general background variables. Several informants had been participating in more than one group activity.

Results

The majority of the participants reported having improved their health status, quality of life, and function, particularly when given the opportunity to utilize their own abilities and creativity, thus increasing their self-efficacy and self-esteem. 78% of the 46 informants were between 40–69 years old. 43% had higher education. 73% had participated or been attached to The NaCuHeal Centre for at least two years. 27 persons were certified as sick during the study. 82% reported problems like stress-symptoms, psychosocial problems, anxiety-depression, muscular-symptoms, tiredness/lack of energy, and sleep-disturbances. Most of these problems were related to work or home situations. If participants had experienced a negative home situation, they would bring these experiences and their difficult life situation with them to work and vice versa. Half of the participants mentioned relational problems and divorce as a major hindrance to a positive life situation. Most participants explained that if they had problems coping in everyday life, their quality of life decreased and so did their health. Most participants used expressions like 'burn-out', 'the last straw', 'batteries had gone flat', 'deflated', or 'hit the wall'. The majority of the participants were particular occupied with the question of why people become so ill and how they could maintain health, obtain a better lifestyle, and/or change health behaviour.

Due to different coping strategies, background, and resources, the informants seemed to be divided into three typical categories. These categories are analyzed according to different variables, like educational background, age, period of participation in group activities, function, and present life situation, problems, and symptoms. These variables have also been analysed in relation to the main focus of the project and to the different themes that appeared through the interviews.

Category 1. The role model: Eleven persons (23%) seemed to fall into this category. They had fairly strong beliefs in the factors which they assumed maintained or developed their own health and quality of life. They thought that they knew what 'a good life is'. Arguing along these lines, one could say that participation in activity groups could maintain or enhance their health and quality of life. These people were resourceful and energetic and had a lot to give to others. In addition, they believed that the interaction between nature and culture had a strong effect on health by giving a new enrichment and spirit to their lives. The participants seemed to function as ambassadors, role models and intermediaries for other participants in their process of improving their health and quality of life. Quote: 'I am happy and satisfied with my life and if I can bring to other people some light and joy, this is a place I would like to support...'

Category 2. Lacking coping strategies: 21 persons (45%) belonged to this category in certain ways. They believed that the NaCuHeal Centre had influenced, inspired, and developed their creative abilities, particularly in relation to painting and music (Small 1998). The participants were resourceful persons, but due to a huge workload, stress, and lack of coping strategies, they had been very ill. Terms like 'deflated', 'the last straw', etc., were particularly apt for those in this group. Life had been too hectic for a long period of time, and without possibilities for relaxation and regaining their energy level, they were unable to prevent illnesses like chronic fatigue, muscular diseases, anxiety, and depression. Through participation in group activities, their self-efficacy and sense of coherence had increased considerably and sometimes to such an extent that the willingness and motivation to go back to work was imminent: Quote: 'Now I feel ready to return to work. I think the society could have saved a lot of money if only people could be given opportunities like this, being at NaCuHeal…'

Category 3. Huge benefits from participating in group activities: 14 persons (30%) seemed to belong to this category. Life had been full of minor or major crises, their health had declined, and one could describe their overall life situation as problematic and complex. Several had limited educational background and were at risk for developing severe and chronic illnesses. Participation in the group activities at NaCuHeal gave many a valuable experience along with good, stable relationships. In addition, the group activities had helped them out of isolation and loneliness. Many of them did not have any social network, or they had been deprived of social contact due to their life situation, e.g. divorce, illnesses, moving, etc. Typical quotes: 'NaCuHeal has meant so much for me. You could say that it has saved my life…'; Quote: 'I don't believe that one can push pills into ones body endlessly. This is much better than all the pills in the whole world. Talk with someone, share knowledge and experience and opinions…'

Evaluation study 2:
Music and Health Promotion. The role and significance of music in everyday life for the long-term ill

The second evaluation study presented here focuses on recent discussions about music and health, while emphasizing a need for qualitative studies with an ethnographic approach. The overall aim of this study was to highlight the way that music can act as a sort of folk-medical practice in our contemporary culture to maintain, improve, or change health status, though it is administered in a non-professional setting (Ruud 2005; Stige 2004). Even though music has been considered as a contributor to our health, music is basically absent from any political, national, or local community discussions about health and quality of life. In several public reports and articles on health promotion and public health in Norway (e.g., White Paper. St. meld. 29 1996–7; White Paper. St. meld. 16 2002–2003), music is hardly mentioned as a contributing factor to health and wellbeing. This evaluation study focused on the beneficial factors of participating in a yearlong project 'Music and Health Promotion', and it discussed the major outcomes and significance of participating in the study, focusing on participants' own subjective opinions and attitudes (Batt-Rawden & Tellnes 2005; Batt-Rawden 2010, 2010a). This study considered how and why outcomes of participation seemed to be linked to increased levels of consciousness and self-awareness, and thus connected to processes of change, care of self, and self-development. Furthermore, it discussed how music can trigger social action and human agency and why this may be linked to health, social network, and quality of life.

There were two aims of the second evaluation study (2)

This study took an exploratory approach, examining an area where there has been little data and building upon previous work that has focused on music, health, and everyday life. There were two main objectives:
1. To explore the role and significance of musicking in the life of men and women with long-term illnesses in different life phases, situations, events, issues, and contexts.
2. To increase knowledge of how participants, through exposure to and exchange of new musical materials and practices, may learn to use music as a 'technology of self' in relation to health and healing; and to do this using a method which involved participation in the design of music CDs.

This focus highlighted 'music education' or informal musical learning, as discussed by Green (2002), specifically individuals' development of skills and knowledge in the use of music for enrichment and coping, and as an instrument of change. This is a technique that can be learnt (as opposed to technologies that exist to produce, compose or disseminate music), such as musicking (Small 1998) as a mental health promotion procedure.

Evaluation methodology

This study included the participants' own subjective opinions, life experiences, and life-worlds, and the main focus was to increase knowledge about the role and significance of music in relation to health, illness, and quality of life in everyday life for men and women with long-term illnesses. This action-oriented research project involved eight in-depth ethnographic interviews and open narratives, with a sample of nine men and thirteen women, aged 35–65 with long-term illnesses or diseases, i.e. muscular disease, chronic fatigue, burnt-out, anxiety and depression, cancer, and neurological disease. It was a longitudinal study stretching over a whole year from 2004 to 2005, including an interactive use of CD listening and choosing. Thirteen people received disability pension or rehabilitation benefits, and two worked part-time. Seven had returned to work, one was a housewife, and one had recovered but was still unemployed.

Results

The typical descriptions of the outcome of participation were an increased self-awareness and consciousness of life-changing issues, events, memories, and habits, in which music had played a key role in their lives. Further, the project had inspired or motivated several to act socially, and this contributed to their sense of wellbeing and a stronger 'care of self'. In other words, they were able to connect body, mind, and spirit to a sense of wholeness through music or musicking and thus act as a technology of the self by regulating the body-mind relationship (DeNora 2000). Participants that had not been conscious of how they used music previously or how music matters seemed to have gained a new perspective and understanding in relation to their musical activities and practices in everyday life, particularly in relation to health and illness.

Music, consciousness and self-awareness

Through partaking in the 'Music and Health Promotion' project, the majority of the participants claimed that it had raised their consciousness and self-awareness about the significance of music in their life and its vital link to health and quality of life. This male participant explained how he had gained self-awareness during this project, how it had changed the focus in his life and how music had helped him in the process of change and self-development:

It has heightened my awareness, doing this project, like reflecting on why in that particular moment in your life, this song means something special to you, what is the connection. Is it something old, or is it something new, or is it something I need?... And how it works for me and how it heals and how it can help me through something or towards something new... Music is a huge well of reservoir of resources... When you learn a new piece of music, it changes your focus in your life, it brings you into the flow of life, so that you can change without resisting the change. (Male nurse, age, 53, recovered from depression before fieldwork started)

The majority of the participants described heightened awareness in terms of feelings about a 'new self', a 'new lifestyle', or new directions for enhancing wellbeing. Another male participant suggested that this method ought to be used for health-promotion in institutions or hospitals, because it increases self-awareness, which triggers reflections and coping strategies concerning difficult life issues and emotions. This participant told how this increased consciousness made him aware of how he uses music to regulate his mood, humour, and state of mind, and he said that it is incredible what music can do. Through such a project, he suggested, one could give people a task to teach them the importance of reflection:

I have started to think more consciously on how I use music, for example, what do I want to listen to today, and then I choose something that corresponds with my mood, humour, emotions, or spirituality... I think it is amazing what music can do...There are so many things I really haven't thought about before and, I think, one should give people a task, which is learning to reflect consciously through such a project. (Male, age, 50, long-term certified sick for two years due to a burnt out. Recovered before fieldwork started)

Evaluation study 3:
The benefits of a holistic and salutogenic approach to rehabilitation and recreation

The third evaluation paper presents result from a study conducted by Eastern Norway Research Institute (ENRI) in collaboration with Fron Rehabilitation Centre, Norway in 2008–2009 (Batt-Rawden & Tellnes 2010). Fron

Rehabilitation Centre takes a salutogenic and holistic view on health that emphasizes physical activity, psychological methods, and nature experiences as pathways to treatment and rehabilitation. Their main objective is to help people to return to work and regain strength, vitality, and energy. During a four-week long stay at Fron Rehabilitation Centre, the participants are offered two sessions of physical activity[3] and nature experiences[4] daily, combined with sessions on energy psychology (Gallo 1998) and tutorials on lifestyle changes, both individually and in groups. The rehabilitation process through four weeks focuses on learning how thoughts, beliefs, actions, relationships, social networks, and environment may influence our energy levels, function, and capacity for work, grounded in the life experiences and current life situation of the participants.

There were three aims of the third evaluation study (3)

1. To evaluate subjective health and wellbeing among participant's at Fron Rehabilitation Centre during four week stay.
2. To increase Fron Rehabilitation Centre's own knowledge about how and why various rehabilitation programmes seem to contribute to perceived benefits for the participants.
3. To evaluate subjective health and wellbeing among participants who were present for the follow-up week at Fron Rehabilitation Centre two months later.

Evaluation methodology

Eastern Norway Research Institute (ENRI) conducted a qualitative (part I and part II) evaluation study in collaboration with Fron Rehabilitation Centre, Norway in 2008–2009. The first part of the study included 38 participants and their subjective opinions, beliefs, and life experiences of being at Fron Rehabilitation Centre during their four week stay. Each participant was interviewed twice: once each during the first and last week. Part two included an in-depth interview with 19 participants, exploring their subjective experiences and outcomes of being a part of the follow-up week two months

---

[3] Physical activities at Fron Rehabilitation Centre include walking, swimming, gym, and dance.
[4] Outdoor activities include walking in the forest, mountains or through cultural landscapes.

later. These participants were selected[5] through a raffle on the last day of the fourth week, i.e. randomly chosen to have the opportunity to participate in the follow-up week. Both parts of the study were conducted using a semi-structured interview guide. Age groups for all participants were 23–60. The participants were suffering from long-term illness, e.g. muscular disease, burn-out, or mental problems and had a low socio-economic background. The interviewer audiotaped the interviews and transcribed them verbatim immediately after the dialogue. The participants were asked to sign an informed consent document. Grounded theory was chosen as the qualitative methodological approach, since the research questions attempted to explore and describe social processes of illness and health as they emerged from the ethnographic data. This method involves a process of coding, categorization, and comparison of the interview data (Charmaz 2003).

Results

The majority of the participants felt that the Fron Rehabilitation Centre had given them a new platform, a renewed way of thinking and reasoning, a repertoire of new skills, and a different way of handling their own actions and behaviour. As one participant expressed it, 'I would recommend this centre to other people whom I know would benefit from staying here. It's fantastic in so many ways, and I have learned a lot'. Typical descriptions were related to stress and mental and physical burdens in everyday life, including pressure to tackle the burdens from an active working career. The majority of the participants had struggled with lack of control over several dimensions in life, like work, caring responsibilities, bad economy, divorce, and lack of opportunities and life chances in general. The majority of the participants described an experienced lack of energy and power, often referring to their own dysfunctional life situation: 'It's just no life and everything is terrible right now, and I am feeling that I can't do anything to control my life situation. And I feel that I am in a state of sorrow... I hope this place can help me to turn the wheel in the right direction', or 'it looks as if everything is tied together, my pain gets worse and worse, and then I get more and more depressed, and then I feel sorry for myself'.

---

[5] Fron Rehabilitation Centre at Hundorp, North of Lillehammer, had been given financial support by the Ministry of Health to try out one follow-up week for the first time in 2008.

Three main factors seemed to contribute to participants' perceived recovery and wellbeing:

(1) Physical activities and nature experience

It seems that outdoor physical activity, like walking in the forest or in the mountains or sitting calmly and looking at the countryside after a brisk walk, and an active lifestyle have a substantial positive effect on wellbeing. Furthermore, being physically active has a positive effect on self-esteem and self-perceptions, including body image: 'I feel much better when I am physically active every day. It gives me energy and vitality, and I don't get so depressed'.

(2) The social environment and Sense of Coherence

An important factor which contributed to participants' sense of being in the process of recovery might have been how the social environment served as a type of significant other, supporting a sense of coherence and predictability (Antonovsky 1987). The environment hence might have given the participants some vitality and energy through meaningful interactions. In this respect, difficult or adverse life circumstances and negative emotions may be modified and transformed via social strategies for achieving a readjustment of the self over time: 'Being here has made me rethink how I live my life, and how I can change my behaviour and live a different life in the future. I will focus on the daily routines I have learned here'.

(3) Learning to adopt a new lifestyle

The participants had increased their self-awareness and consciousness about the importance of physical activity, and this awareness contributed to feelings of wellbeing and vitality. Through learning new techniques, the participants' energy was channeled into action and lifestyle changes, which helped to maintain good health habits: 'I have learned so many new ways of thinking and acting, but it is also important to have the opportunity to come back and repeat what we have learned, since it is so easy to forget or even get back to old habits again when your're home'.

The follow-up week two months later

Most participants perceived a further improvement in their and health and wellbeing after they joined the follow-up week. Through re-learning and repeating new techniques, the participants' adopted lifestyle became a coping strategy and a way of performing physical and mental healing and maintaining good health habits. Typical descriptions from the follow-up week were: 'Generally speaking, I feel much better now' or 'The follow-up week has made me rethink my life situation, and they have guided me in the right direction' or 'It is good to know that you are working with yourself rightly, you know, and this week has only confirmed I am on the right path'.

General discussion

A Holistic Nature-Culture-Health approach includes a salutogenic perspective

These three studies employ a holistic approach to health, sickness absence, rehabilitation, and recovery, and this approach includes a salutogentic perspective (Antonovsky 1987; Lindstrøm & Ericsson 2005; Suominen & Lindstrøm 2008; Tellnes 2009). This perspective focuses on how one may reach new and better constructions of meaning to attain ontological security and the processes by which this is achieved, both unconsciously and consciously (Giddens 1991). The findings in these evaluation studies support recent studies which conclude that active participation in cultural, physical, and recreational activities reduces pain and anxiety, promotes health, and increases longevity (Knudtsen, Holmen & Håpnes 2005; Ruud 2002). Illness is a disruption not only of structures of explanation and meaning but also of the sustenance of normal relationships and of the mobilization of resources (Bury 1982). Thus, monitoring illness using a holistic approach may increase self-knowledge and awareness, which in turn might give individuals a sense of coping that might help them to move on in their process of recovery. Health problems are connected to the whole person, and it may be difficult to determine the contribution of different parts. Social problems in private life may influence our health situation, and the social situation in our work place may improve or worsen the situation (Tellnes 1990). As Sewell (1992) argues, part of what it means to conceive of human beings as agents is to conceive of them as empowered by access to resources of one kind or another. For example, the Fron Rehabilitation Centre and the NaCuHeal Centre seem to support and help those agents who are capable of putting their structurally formed capacities to work in creative or innovative ways. A person has to believe that when starting a task, one has to complete it with success. There is no other way apart from saying: 'I am capable of doing this'.

Through participation in Nature-Culture-Health activities, hidden resources and creativity are awakened. Participants feel good about themselves and what they do is appreciated. In this way, one can strengthen the salutogenetic factors in a person's life (Antonovsky 1987). In other words, by focusing on promoting health factors, one might actually promote health in the process (Laverack 2004; Tones & Green 2004). From this perspective, a holistic Nature-Culture-Health approach would consider the whole life situation of a person in order to understand the complexities involved in sickness absence (Tellnes 2009). Engaging in daily routines involving different activities at the NaCuHeal Centre, in the 'Music and Health Promotion' study and at Fron Rehabilitation centre, the majority of participants from all three studies experienced a sense of coherence (Eriksson & Lindstrøm 2006; Antonovsky 1987). This coherence had direct physiological and psychological consequences, affecting their health status (Suominen & Lindstrøm 2008), particularly in coping with stressors in everyday life or through the rehabilitation process (Griffiths 2009). Previous studies also show correlations between sense of coherence and mental health and wellbeing (Langius & Bjorvell 1993; Eriksson 2009). This sense of coherence perspective common to these three studies seems to help people to strengthen their resilience and to develop a positive subjective state of health.

Music, consciousness and self-awareness

The Music and Health Promotion project might teach participants how to use music, thus triggering memories and raising levels of consciousness. It gives participants a feeling of happiness and inspires them to search for new music or musicking that opens up for self-reflection, self-reflexivity, self-development, emotional competence, and social action. Through musical memories, a new relationship between past and present seems to be forged. Music provides a sense of being included in a 'larger than life' context (Gouk 2000), and significant life events and situations may be regarded in a different light and be given a new meaning, thus increasing self-awareness. (Charmaz 1991; 1999). Musical narratives also seem to play a vital role in the participant's everyday life relating to memories of happy times and of meaningful moments. Frith (2003) argues that musical experiences open up for a kind of self-consciousness, a coming together of the sensual, the emotional, and the social through performance. Music constructs our sense of identity through the experiences of the body, time, and sociability, and these experiences enable us to place ourselves in imaginative cultural narratives. DeNora (2000) discusses how music creates an emotional and cognitive context that is conducive to a feeling of wellbeing and a state of alertness or relaxation in accordance with the needs of the situation. Music is present in a variety of social and personal contexts where mood is regulated, attention focused, and energy channeled. Music can be used as a device for the reflexive process of remembering and constructing who one is, a technology for spinning the apparently continuous tale of is the *self*. This notion connects to the development of a strong self and a sense of meaning.

By emphasizing a salutogenetic perspective through empowerment and participation among different groups of the population (those with illness and disease or people at risk or other life complications and problems), the mediators need no professional knowledge or competence in music itself. One could stimulate follow-up musical activities using health professionals as mediators, by building social networks outside the hospital and primary health-care settings, whereby people could engage in musical activities in local communities. The participants can then initiate music appreciation groups, go to concerts together, sing or play together, i.e. musicking (Small. 1998), without the help of health professionals. They could thus shape culture through weaving musically and stimulating close networks. Individuals are bound together through common social experiences, and they thus establish a meeting place where they can have a sense of belonging.

Final comments

Results from these evaluation studies indicate how art, music, and nature-culture-health activities may have a beneficial impact on health and wellbeing, and hence be useful for rehabilitation. It is important to continue to stimulate the refinement, focus, and implementation of future health-promotion and rehabilitation programs in interdisciplinary cooperation. Nature-culture-health experiences may help the participants to construct a meaning, to identify coping mechanisms, and to revitalize the energetic and resourceful parts of the self. Moreover, the salutogenic approach could create a solid theoretical framework for health promotion (Eriksson & Lindstrøm

2006; 2008; Suominen & Lindstrøm 2008), and it may counteract events leading to sickness absence (Eriksson 2009). For example, according to these authors, burnout might be understood as a process of emotional deprivation, whereby the individual is gradually emptied of the life-giving emotional energy that is expressed as joy, commitment, and empathy.

Synthetic research methods probably have to be applied in order to evaluate the community approach to public health used at the NaCuHeal centres. Our experience is that Nature-Culture-Health activities can help us promote the public's environment, health and quality of life, and that they would be worth implementing more widely than they are today (Batt-Rawden & Tellnes 2005; Tellnes 2004; 2009).

References

Aldridge, D. 1996. *Music Therapy Research and Practices in Medicine. From out of Silence.* London, Jessica Kingsley Publishers

Alexanderson, K. 2005. 'Research on sickness absence and disability pension'. Tellnes, G. ed.: *Urbanization and Health. New challenges to Health Promotion and Prevention.* Oslo, Unipub (Oslo Academic Press)

Antonovsky, A. 1987. *Unravelling the Mystery of Health.* San Fransisco, Jossey-Bass

Batt-Rawden, K.B. & Tellnes, G. 2005. 'Nature-Culture-Health Activities as a Method of Rehabilitation: An Evaluation of Participants' Health, Quality of Life and Function'. *International Journal of Rehabilitation Research.* Vol 28 (2), 175–180

Batt-Rawden, K.B. & Tellnes, G. 2005a. 'Music and Health Promotion. A case study'. Tellnes, G. ed.: *Urbanization and Health. New challenges to Health Promotion and Prevention.* Oslo, Unipub (Oslo Academic Press)

Batt-Rawden, K.B., DeNora, T. & Ruud, E. 2005. 'Music Listening and Empowerment in Health Promotion: A study of the Role and Significance of Music in Everyday Life of the Long-term Ill'. *Nordic Journal of Music Therapy.* Vol 14 (2), 120–136

Batt-Rawden, K.B. & DeNora, T. 2005. 'Music and Informal Learning in Everyday Life'. *Music Education Research*, Vol. 7 (3), 289–304

Batt-Rawden, K.B., & Tellnes, G. 2010. 'The benefits of a holistic and salutogenic approach to rehabilitation and recreation'. Kofler, W. & Khalilov, E. eds.: *Science without Borders*. Special Edition, 103–111

Batt-Rawden, K.B. 2010. 'Music as a technology of health and well-being'. *International Journal of Mental Health Promotion*. Volume 12, Issue 2, 11–18

Batt-Rawden, K.B. 2010a. 'The benefits of self-selected music on health and well being'. *The Arts in Psychotherapy*. In press

Blaxter, M. 2000. 'Class, time and biography'. Williams, S.J., Gabe, J. & Calnan, M. eds.: *Health, Medicine and Society: Key Theories, Future Agendas*. London, Routledge.

Bury M. 1982. 'Chronic illness as biographical disruption'. *Sociology of Health and Illness*. 4 (2), 167–82

Charmaz, K. 1991. *Good Days, Bad Days. The Self in Chronic Illness and Time*. New Brunswick, New Jersey, Rutgers University Press

Charmaz, K. 1999. 'Stories of Suffering: Subjective Tales and Research. Narratives'. In: *Qualitative Health Research*. Vol 9 (3). London, Sage Publications, 362–382

Charmaz K. 2003. 'Grounded Theory'. Smith, J.A. ed.: *Qualitative Psychology. A Practical Guide to Research Methods*. London, Sage Publications

Conrad, P. 1987. 'The experience of illness'. *Research in the Sociology of Health Care,* 61–31

Crawford, R. 2000. 'The ritual of health promotion'. Williams, S.J, Gabe, J. & Calnan, M. eds.: *Health, Medicine and Society: Key Theories, Future Agendas*. London, Routledge

DeNora, T. 2000. *Music in Everyday Life*. Cambridge, Cambridge University Press

Eriksson M. & Lindström B. 2008. 'Promoting mental health - Evidence of the salutogenic framework for a positive health development'. *Eur Psychiatry.* 23 (Suppl. 2)

Eriksson M. & Lindström B. 2006. 'Antonovsky's sense of coherence scale and the relation with health: a systematic review'. *J Epid Com Health*. 2: 60, 376–381. http://jech.bmjournals.com

Eriksson U.B. 2009. 'After all you're only human- Long-term sickness absence from emotional, relational and structural perspectives'. PhD-thesis. Karlstad, Sweden, Karlstad University Studies

Frith, S. 2003. 'Music and Everyday Life'. Clayton, M., Herbert, T. & Middelton R. eds.: *The Cultural Study of Music. A Critical Introduction*. New York, Routledge, 92–101

Gallo F.P. 1998. *Energy psychology: explorations at the interface of energy, cognition, behaviour, and health*. Pennsylvania, Boca Raton, CRC Press

Gerhardt, U. 2000. 'Narratives of normality: End-stage renal-failure patients' experience of their transplant options'. Williams, S.J., Gabe, J. & Calnan, M. eds.: *Health, Medicine and Society: Key Theories, guture agendas*. London, Routledge

Giddens A. 1991. *Modernity and Self-Identity*. Cambridge, Polity Press

Green, L. 2002. *How Popular Musicians Learn. A way ahead for music education*. Aldershot, Ashgate

Griffiths C.A. 2009. 'Sense of coherence and mental rehabilitation'. *Clin Rehabil*: 23 (1), 72–8

Goffman, E. 1961. *Asylums. Essays on the social situation of mental patients and other inmates*. Penguin Books

Gouk, P. 2000. *Musical Healing in Cultural Contexts*. Aldershot, Ashgate

Holmboe-Ottesen, G. & Tellnes, G. 2005. 'Urbanisation and public health challenges in Europe'. Tellnes, G. ed.: *Urbanization and Health. New Challenges to Health Promotion and Prevention*. Oslo, Unipub (Oslo Academic Press).

Karaberg, D., Tellnes, G. & Karaberg A. 2004. 'NaCuHeal Information Design in Public Health: Synthetic Research Models of the Nature-Culture-Health Interplay'. *Michael* 1, 247–51

Konlaan, B.B. 2001. *Cultural Experience and Health: The Coherence of Health and Leisure Time Activities*. Umeå, University Medical Dissertations

Konlaan, B.B., Bygren, L.O. & Johansson, S-E. 2000. 'Visiting cinema, concerts, museums or art, exhibitions as dominant of survival: a Swedish fourteen-year cohort follow up'. *Scand J Public Health*. Vol 28 (3) ,174–178

Knudtsen, M.S., Holmen, J. & Håpnes, O. 2005. 'Kulturelle virkemidler i behandling og folkehelsearbeid' (Culture used in therapy and public health). *Tidsskr Nor Lægeforen* 125, 3434–6. In Norwegian. English summary

Langius A. Bjorvell H. 1993. 'Coping ability and functional status in a Swedish population sample'. *Scand J Caring*. 7 (1), 3–10

Laverack, G. 2004. *Health Promotion Practice: Power and Empowerment*. London, Sage Publications

Lindstrøm, B. & Eriksson, M. 2005. 'Salutogenesis'. *J. Epidemiol. Community Health* Vol 59 (6), 440–442

Naidoo, J. & Wills, J. 2000. *Health Promotion*. London, Bailliere Tindall.

Noack, H. R. 2005. 'Building the Modern Public Health: Perspectives, Theory and Practice'. Tellnes, G. ed.: *Urbanization and Health. New challenges to Health Promotion and Prevention*. Oslo, Unipub (Oslo Academic Press)

Pausewang, E. 1999. Organizing Modern Longings. Paradoxes in the construction of a health promotive community in Norway. Thesis. Oslo, University of Oslo, Institute of Social Anthropology

Radley, A. 1997. 'What role does the body have in illness?' Yardely, L. ed.: *Material Discourses of Health and Illness*. London, Routledge

Ruud, E. 2002. 'Music as a Cultural Immunogen – Three Narratives on the Use of Music as a Technology of Health'. Hanken, I.M., Nilsen, S.G. & Nerland, M. eds.: *Research in and for Higher Music Education. Festschrift for Harald Jøregensen*. Oslo, NMH-Publications, 2002: 2

Ruud, E. 2005. *Lydlandskap. Om bruk og misbruk av musikk*. [Soundscapes. About Use and Misuse of Music]. Bergen, Norway, Fagbokforlaget

Rønning R., Batt-Rawden K.B., Solheim, L. 2008. *Care work and sickness absence*. Report ENRI 2009/1. Lillehammer, East Norwegian Research Institute

Savage, J. 2005. 'Sound2Picture: developing compositional pedagogies from the sound designer's world'. *Music Education Research*. Vol 7 (3), 331–348

Sewell W.H 1992. 'A theory of structure: duality, agency, and transformation'. *AmJ Sociology*: 98 (1), 1–29

Small, C. 1998. *Musicking. The Meanings of Performing and Listening*. London, Welsyan Press

Stige, B. 2004. 'Community Music Therapy: Culture, Care and Welfare'. Pavlicevic, M. & Ansdell, G. eds.: *Community Music Therapy*. London and Philadelphia, Jessica Kingsley Publishers

Stige, B. 2005. 'Music as a health resource'. *Nordic Journal of Music Therapy*. 14 (1).http://www.hisf.no/njmt/editorial141.html (retrieved online 2nd of November, 2005)

Suominen S. & Lindstrøm B. 2008. 'Salutogenese'. *Scand J Public Health* 36, 337–9

Tellnes, G. 1990. Sickness certification – an epidemiological study related to community medicine and general practice. Dissertation. Oslo, University of Oslo, Department of Community Medicine

Tellnes, G. 1996. 'Integration of Nature-Culture-Health as a method of prevention and rehabilitation'. In UNESCOs Report from the International Conference on Culture and Health, Oslo, Sept. 1995. Oslo, The Norwegian National Committee of the World Decade for Cultural Development

Tellnes, G. 2003. 'Public Health and the Way Forward'. Kirch, W. ed.: *Public Health in Europe*. Berlin, Springer-Verlag

Tellnes, G. 2003a. *Samspillet Natur-Kultur-Helse.* [The Nature-Culture-Health Interplay] Oslo, Unipub (Oslo Academic Press)

Tellnes, G. 2004. 'The Community Approach to Public Health'. *Michael* 1, 206–11

Tellnes G. 2009. 'How can nature and culture promote health?' *Scand J Public Health*. 37, 559–561

Tones, K. & Green, J. 2004. *Health Promotion; Planning and Strategies.* London, Sage Publications

White Paper. NOU 1998: 18. Det er bruk for alle. [We need everyone]. Oslo, The Government of Norway

White Paper. St. Meld. Nr. 16. 2002–2003. Resept for et sunnere Norge. [A recipe for a Healthier Norway]. Oslo, The Government of Norway

White Paper. St. Meld. 29 1996–7. Utfordringer i helsefremmende og forebyggende arbeid. [Challenges in Public Health and Health Promotion]. Oslo, The Government of Norway

Williams, S. J., Gabe, J. & Calnan, M. eds. 2000. *Health, Medicine and Society: Key Theories, Future Agendas.* London, Routledge

Chapter 13

Helpers of the fragile, elderly and sick: Report from a nursing home

Kari Batt-Rawden & Liv Johanne Solheim

Summary

In the past few years, health and social services has been one of the branches with the highest percentage of its employees certified as sick. This chapter focuses on a part of this branch, presenting a case study on sickness absence among employees in a nursing home. There are two objectives in this study: first, the individuals' experiences of their working situation along with their own views of the causes of their sickness absence and, second, the individuals' experiences of the role of being certified as sick. The employees described negative changes in the working conditions during the last years. A major finding is that work overload seems to be the dominant reason for sickness absence, though, for some, a problem in the private sphere was the determining factor. The role of being certified as sick influenced the participants' identity and made them vulnerable to being stigmatized.

Introduction

Statistics show that sickness absence varies among different branches, and that health and social services has recently been one of the branches with the highest percentage of its employees certified as sick (www.nav.no/243644.

cms). This chapter focuses on a part of this branch, presenting a case study about sickness absence among employees in a nursing home (Rønning et al. 2009). One of the general characteristics in nursing homes is that the majority of the employees are women. Another is that there is relational and emotional work at these institutions. During the last decades, there has been a transformation of the tasks in working life from production-oriented to relational and emotional work (Forseth 2001). According to Hochshild (1983, 147), emotional work is characterized by three components: face to face or voice to voice contact with the public, the worker's production of an emotional state in another person, and the employer's exercise, through training and supervision, of a degree of control over emotional activities of employees. Examples of professional groups engaged in emotional work are teachers, social workers, nurses, and care workers. These kinds of professional groups are vulnerable to different kinds of problems if the employees are not able to handle the emotions they activate in their clients, and these problems may influence sickness absence.

In order to understand social factors influencing sickness absence, it is also important to consider how sickness absence identities are created as a function of the social interaction between those who are certified as sick and their social networks. A person may have health problem without sickness absence or, conversely, sickness absence without illness or disease. In this way, some people may assume no sick role even when they have an illness or a disease, for example, those who continue their work as usual without receiving a sickness certificate (Tellnes 1990). Some social networks may also be more willing to accept different forms of sickness absence than others.

We approach understanding the phenomenon of sickness absence with two considerations in mind. First, factors in a person's work situation as well as his or her private sphere may influence health problems as well as sickness absence. Second, a sickness absence identity is created as a function of the social interaction between those who are certified as sick and their social network. In this chapter, we give a presentation of the persons' own views of the causes of their sickness absence (a 'total situation' approach), and we give their descriptions of the role of being certified as sick, of general attitudes towards those who are sickness absent, and of how they feel they are treated.

Current research on sickness absence in emotional work

A report on the current state of knowledge on sickness absence, made for The Research Council of Norway (Ose et al. 2006), mentions social factors several times (gender, life-style etc.) but lacks an explicit discussion of them. This fact reflects the situation of the scientific discussion on sickness absence: social factors are broadly accepted as being important, but they are seldom mentioned as a main focus. There is considerable research on the relationship between the psychosocial conditions in working life in general and sickness absence in particular. In their survey of research on the effect of working conditions on mental health problems and sickness absence, Michi and Williams (2003) have found that several factors were critical: long hours, excessive work under pressure, lack of opportunities to influence one's work situation, and poor support from managers. This research supports earlier findings about the significance of social support (e.g. Siegrist 1996). Several studies find that reorganisation and downsizing increases the chances for burnout (Vahtera et al. 2004; Verhaeghe et al. 2003; Hallsten & Isaksson 2001). Eriksson (2009) has described the road to sickness absence as a step-by-step process and presents a burnout staircase with eight steps (see also Eriksson et al., chapter 8). Eriksson (2009) found that the role of being certified as sick seems to be a process of emotional deprivation, resulting in serious psychosomatic health problems.

A review of the research literature has shown that emotional work has both negative and positive effects on health problems (Kruml & Geddes 2000). The reported negative consequences were burnout, stress, depression, and low self-confidence. Examples of positive effects were: satisfaction, self-confidence, low stress level, and mental well-being. It is also important to make a distinction between positive and negative stress (Eriksson 2009). Positive stress is defined as inner tension, which the individual experiences as positive. Negative stress occurs when there is incongruence between the external demands and the individuals' needs and abilities. Social, cultural, and economic aspects may influence what individuals experience as stress. Some researchers have moved from talking about burnout on an individual level to burnout in connection with organisations (Maslach & Leiter 1997).

This may be a relevant characteristic of sections of the health and social services branch, especially in care for elderly, because there has been an increasing demand for services in this field without a corresponding extension of the capacity. The consequence has been strong pressure on the employees in facilities for elderly people as well as on those working in home care. This is a situation in which the employees are vulnerable for being certified as sick, thus potentially increasing the level of sickness absence. However, health problems and sickness absence may have causes other than the work situation. A study based upon data across branches showed that about 50% of the episodes of sickness absence lasting more than two weeks were related to the work situation (Olsen 2007). During the last few years, there have been extensive changes in both private and public enterprises. Some of these changes are: reorganisations, increasing demands for qualitative and quantitative flexibility, outsourcing of employees and entities, fusions, and network- and project-organizing. Psychosocial demands at the workplace may give rise to conflicts between employees (Schabraq, 2003). Norwegian workplaces have also been influenced by this development, but the effect on sickness absence is still unclear (Gamperiene et al. 2007, 25).

Theoretical perspectives

Karasek and Theorell (1990) presented a model for describing the connection between demand and control in one's work environment. They argue that the combination of high demands in the workplace and limited possibilities to decide how and when work is performed leads to increasing stress levels, resulting in negative health consequences. They also show that support in one's work environment can be an important buffer against this combination. In the following, we describe this model in more detail (see also Engström & Eriksson 2010, chapter 10).

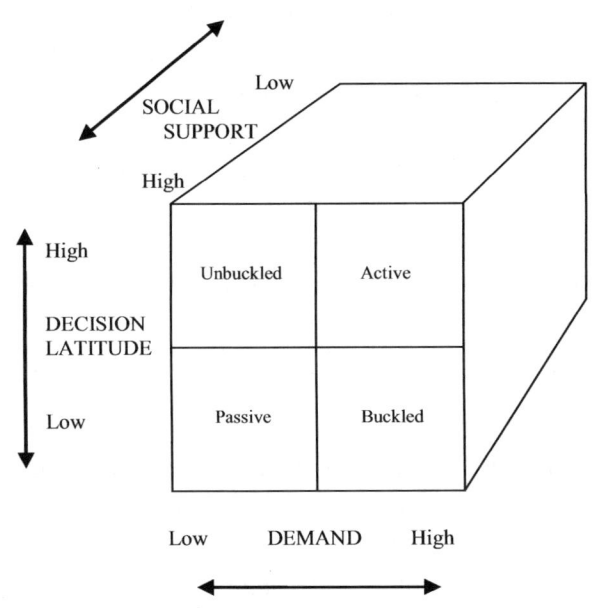

Figur 1: Demand – control – social support model.

The first dimension refers to the demands placed on employees, including demands for efficiency and emotional and cognitive demands. The second dimension refers to decision latitude, or the possibilities for employees to control their own working situation. One aspect of decision latitude is decision authority, which refers to the opportunities the organisation provides for a worker to decide how to do his or her job. Another aspect is the control over the skills and development of competence, or so-called skill discretion. The basic idea behind this model is that the balance between mental demands and decision latitude has a decisive influence on an employee's working situation. High psychological demands are supposed to promote sickness only if there are few possibilities to influence the situation. The combination of high mental demands and low decision latitude is called 'buckled work', while high mental demands combined with high decision latitude is called 'active work'. Low mental demands in combination with low decision latitude are called 'passive work', and low mental demands combined with high decision latitude are called 'unbuckled work'. The different situations result in differing long-term effects. The 'buckled work' [tense] will, according to this model, result in an accumulated tension, which makes development and learning difficult. This leads to psychosomatic tensions and increases the risk for sickness absence. In 'active work', it is possible to manage different challenges and to improve coping capabilities. By contrast, the 'passive' position may be described as involving a low mental burden. A consequence of the combination of low demand and low decision latitude is that knowledge and competence is lost. The 'unbuckled' position is supposed to be the ideal working situation (Karasek & Theorell 1990). The third dimension in this the model is social support, or the social climate. In the working environment, the social support from colleagues and superiors is important. Both decision latitude and social support are functions of the work organisation, and, in the modern-day companies, these aspects may be easier to influence than the demand dimension, which often is influenced by external factors.

To understand sickness absence, it is also important to know the general attitudes towards different diagnoses, what reactions people on sickness absence expect from their social network, and how the sickness absent experience the reactions. Sickness absence gives one certain rights (i.e. sickness benefits), has an explanatory function, and creates an identity (Nordby 2004). The person's own capabilities and interpretation of the situation, as well as the reactions from the network, may also be important. Crossley (2001) discusses how individual identities are influenced by the categorizations made by those in one's environment, and how the expectations of the surrounding people influence one's ways of proceeding, actions, and attitudes. Crossley argues that identities are formed within a limited frame of reference. Even when the individuals engage in self-reflection, this reflexivity is mirrored in the collective representations of the society. The social environment is powerful in categorizing individuals and judging their ways of proceeding on the basis of stereotypes. Changes in group norms may be possible, but this will only happen slowly and gradually. What promotes changes in the collective representations is 'the innovate praxis of the agent' (Crossley 2001, 112), that is, the actions of the individuals.

In order to understand the phenomenon of coping, we shall take Antonovsky's (1987; 1996) 'salutogenetic research' as a starting point. He sought to explain connections between health and how we cope with life. Antonovsky sought to trace the general resources of resistance against disease among individuals by identifying coping mechanisms as an instrument of change in difficult life situations. Furthermore, an important factor for health, which Antonovsky labels a 'sense of coherence' (SOC), involves the three aspects: understanding, managing, and making sense of change. A salutogenetic approach to health in times of illness may help an individual to construct meaning or to identify coping mechanisms – a kind of self-reconciliation. This theme relates to the notion that the study of social capital requires conceptual and methodological analyses at an aggregate level, such as in neighbourhoods or small communities, in order to understand satisfactorily its effects on health outcomes (Drentea & Moren-Cross 2005).

Background and aims of the study

Due to high increase in sickness absence at a local nursing home, the institution initiated collaboration with Eastern Norway Research Institute (ENRI) and Lillehammer University College in the autumn of 2008. The employees' long-term sickness absence and the interplay between private and work obligations might have been an influential factor. Long-term sickness absence was defined as having been certified as sick for more than 28 days in a row during the past year; 60 employees belonged to this category. We included both those who had returned to work and those who were still certified as sick at the time of the interviews.

There were two objectives in this study: to investigate and explore individuals' experiences of their working situation and their views of the causes of their sickness absence, and to investigate and explore the individuals' experiences of the role of being long-term certified as sick.

Methods

The study can be described as a case study. Thus, our research strategy involved an empirical and explorative investigation of a phenomenon, in this case, sickness absence at a local nursing home. We selected an explorative design because we wanted to get a better apprehension of the sick absentees' life worlds and of their own understandings of their situation. Qualitative research interviews also provide a way to understand the world from the perspective of the interviewee and to develop the meaning of the individual's experiences (Kvale 1996). We employed open-ended questions to encourage the participants to use their own words to talk about the themes included in the interview guide. The interviewer did use the guide as a list to ensure that every theme had been covered in the interview. The interviews lasted for about 45–90 minutes.

Fifteen (n=15) individuals participated in this study, ranging from 41–65 years old, holding positions as nurses (n=6), as nurse-assistants (n=5), and as non-professionals (n=4). The sample can be described as a convenience sample, that is, one based on the willingness and motivation of participants to dedicate time and effort to the project. Twelve (n=12) of the participants had worked in the health and social services branch for more than 10 years. Only two of the participants had worked at the nursing home for less than five years.

All participants received information about the project verbally and in written form at the onset of the fieldwork. It was stressed that participation was voluntary. Before the interviews, all participants were informed about full confidentiality and about their right to break off participation at any time. The participants were asked to sign a written consent document.

Results

In the following, we first present the participants experiences of their working situation and how they describe the connection between their working situation and their sickness absence. Second, we will give a presentation of their experiences of the role of being long-term certified as sick.

Working situation and the causes of sickness absence

Musculoskeletal problems are a heterogeneous category, covering everything from a broken back to diffuse muscle pain. The majority of the participants in our study either suffered from pains in the neck and shoulders or had headaches. Some also had mental problems, like depression. A few had other diagnoses, like cancer or a broken leg.

The participants' long working experience in this nursing home could be interpreted as an indication of enjoyment in their work, and our study confirmed this to a certain degree. Most of them were dedicated to their work, and twelve participants explicit expressed enjoyment in the challenges connected to their relational work with the elderly people and in the co-operation with their colleagues. However, the majority of the participants were able to describe factors that constitute difficult working conditions and how these factors influenced health and well-being. Most of the participants described negative changes in the working conditions during the last years: more tasks within the same time schedule, more demanding and sick patients, less time for the patients, more kitchen and cleaning work, more demands for documentation, and, in some places, incompetent and absent leadership. In Karasek and Theorell's (1990) vocabulary, their work situation had developed from being unbuckled to tense. This change influenced the employees' work situation and well-being, and for some of them, increasing burdens over time resulted in being certified as sick.

The demands for being more efficient affected their control over their own working situation. Two of them described it like this:

> Yes, there are more hard days now than before, and I am more stressed because of all things I should have done and all tasks that are not done because many are certified as sick.

> ... Earlier the patients were healthier. Now only one of the patients is able to use his own legs. One consequences of this is an increasingly demanding work situation. Nowadays – we never go outside with the patients; there is no time for this... There has been an extraordinary change during the last seven years... We have to do the best we can, but they cut all the way into our soul.

Another aspect of the changes was the demand from those running the organisation that care workers take more responsibility for cleaning and administrative tasks. This demand came at a time when the work with the patients was more time-consuming than ever, and it was not even offset by more hands doing the work. In this way, the nurses and nurse-assistants lost some control over how to spend their time and how to prioritise the patients. They described the working situation as more stressful and less meaningful, since it was impossible to use as much time with the elderly patients as they wanted and as the elderly needed:

> ... I do not like to wash wardrobes and closets when the patients are there and need help... Now the order is that we are going to use even more time on

washing. And the message is to economize with everything – soap, gloves, using fewer handkerchiefs…

The increasing demands and decreasing control over the work created a heavy burden and influenced both their enjoyment of the work situation and their health and sickness absence. One expressed her frustration in this way:

> Yes, I think the economizing affects the enjoyment in one's work. When you get older, you get a better understanding of the situation of elderly people. I can see that they are in need of much help, but I am not able to give them the help they need.

For a few, these experiences had led to reflections on applying for another job. One of these said:

> I do not think I'm going to stay here for a long time. It is totally wrong to go home with bad conscience on behalf of the patients. This is not right! I hope it will be better!… Often you are alone with one patient, and that can be very demanding…

However, for most of them, the positive aspects of the job overshadowed the negative aspects:

> I enjoy the work – I like to be together with the patients with dementia. They have much to tell. They remember things from their past. It is only recent incidents that they do not remember.

One important dimension for care workers is the social support from their colleagues:

> We keep together and we agree – mainly! What we need in these times of economizing is some compliments. We do not get this from the managers, but we praise each other. We know each other very well. Our working conditions and environment function very well.

> … We have been unfortunate with our manager. He is not coping with his tasks, and the consequence is discontent and frustration. But I have excellent colleagues. That is important.

The interviews give a picture of a working situation that over time has become too demanding and stressful for many of the employees. The consequence is musculoskeletal health problems and symptoms of depression and anxiety. However, for some, the explanation of the problems is not to be found only in their working situation, but rather in their private life situation, and for some participants, problems in their private sphere are the determining factors:

> I have had the responsibility for my sick dad who recently died. This happened during a very busy time in my job at the nursing home.

> I have a multi-handicapped daughter at home. This is very wearying, and I feel I never have leisure time.

> I am burned out after too much responsibility at home and in my job.

Some claim that they are tired and need to refuel and to re-energize in order to recover. Personal obligations and duties, like caring for elderly relations, children, or even children with a disability, seem to add to the participants' perception of being under constant pressure with little or no time for leisurely activities. These issues create a picture of a burdened total life situation, with participants often describing how they feel 'burn-out' or 'deflated' due to excessive responsibilities at home and at work. In other words, working conditions and private life burdens seems to have an impact on the development of illness and sickness absence, thus reinforcing the perception of a burdened total life situation. Several complicating factors both privately and work-wise may lead to a continuously stressful situation. It seems almost impossible to regain strength and vitality to function in everyday life, when the opportunity to fulfil such needs is totally absent. A typical quote:

> I am in a very bad shape, and I think I need time to recover… I have been so active and energetic for so many years, and it's not me, really, to be ill like this, but now the cup is full… I have pain in my neck and my back. My doctor said I should try to take it easier and start to exercise more… I have no idea when I will be able to work again…

The role of being certified as sick and constructions of identities.

Our interviews show that the role of being certified as sick is, for many, a difficult position. Some problems, like pain, burnout, loss of initiative, etc., are connected to their health situation. For some participants, it is a lonely situation to be in, especially for those who are living alone. An additionally burden is the relationship to the social surroundings and, in particular, feelings of being stigmatised. The majority of the respondents believe that it is fairly difficult to be accepted in the society when they are long-term certified as sick. However, there are nuances to this assessment, since some diagnoses are considered more acceptable than others.

Some participants think it is a burdensome to have the role of being sick and to be certified as such, and several participants feel that people look at them in a suspicious manner. Several participants believe that the power of other people's views, norms, and beliefs negatively influences their well-being and only adds to a difficult life situation. This was expressed in their hesitation to frequent the places they used to when they were healthy and productive, thereby limiting their personal freedom and space:

> It was a really strange situation; I didn't know what to do with myself... I didn't dare to go out, or to walk around in the town. I was afraid I was going to meet my boss, making him wonder how I could walk around in town while being certified as sick.

> Yes, it was a strange situation. I didn't dare to go out, didn't dare to go into town, since I might meet someone...

> When you are certified as sick you are expected to be invisible.

Very few mentioned explicitly negative reactions towards themselves during the period when they were certified as sick. Their hesitation to go outdoors is, therefore, based upon suspicion, but it may also be influenced by their knowledge about general attitudes towards sickness absence. Moreover, it may also be understood as an expression of their vulnerability and their fear of being stigmatised. Several participants were afraid of meeting people who would suspect them not to be 'rightly' certified as sick or ill. They were afraid of being asked questions about their life situation:

> I do not go through the main street anymore because I'm afraid of meeting people asking why I am sick and their comments that I do not look sick.

This aversion to going out may have been an indication of their vulnerability and feelings of guilt, in the sense that they felt disintegrated and shut out from a successful working life and were coping by trying to reduce the risk of a very unpleasant encounter and, with it, the fear of what might happen. The role of being certified as sick influenced the participants' identity, and the idea of not being able to work and not being healthy or normal reduced their ability to partake in normal daily activities. This, in turn, seemed to increase the chances for developing mental problems, like depression. As one participant said, 'I have had this problem in many years, and right now I have a lot of pain'.

Some participants felt they had lost control over their life situation, contributing to weakening social ties. Single persons are particularly vulnerable:

> By the way, I am becoming very socially isolated since I am single. Also my economic situation is a huge burden. Right now I haven't slept for two nights. I am worried about my economy and my future and everything is like a big black hole. I feel I can't control my own future, things just happen...

However, only a couple of our respondents explicitly claimed that they wanted to keep a distance from their working place during the sickness absence period. Some of them had visited the workplace several times. They said they went there to visit colleagues and patients because they missed them. They experienced that both colleagues and patients appreciated their visits. Here is one example:

> I went there to keep myself updated about what happened and who was doing my jobs. Besides that, I am fond of the elderly people so I want to see them. I was there at least once a week chatting. I missed my workplace – both patients and colleagues.

The caring attitude towards colleagues and patients, displayed even when participants were sickness absent, showed that they have a strong emotional connection to their colleagues and patients. The workplace was, for these participants, an important network and arena for inclusion during their sickness absence. Some participants even described it as a place where they were met by acceptance and understanding:

> There is general understanding for my burnout, and they have contributed to my understanding of the reasons that I have been driven into a corner, a kind of a time trap... All of them know about my history, and I have nothing to hide.

Discussion

Methodological considerations

The research data needs to be put in context. In qualitative studies, it is important to reflect on and consider the role of the researcher: even in action-oriented research projects, 'the observer effect', i.e. the researchers' gender, age and personal characteristics, needs to be taken into account (Schensul et al. 1999). An aspect worth considering is whether these results would have been comparable if someone else had conducted the research.

In line with a qualitative approach, any conclusions drawn from the participants cannot be generalized to the population as a whole. In this sense, our sample is not statistically representative; nevertheless, some tentative general conclusions or final comments may be proposed. We believe that the participants' expressed beliefs and opinions were genuine and real, in relation to how they described their life situations and events during their sickness absence. Even though our study is based upon data from only one nursing home, the situation characterized by increasing demands for services without a corresponding extension of the capacity to meet these demands is well known, both in the nursing homes and in home care in Norway. It may therefore be possible to understand some general tendencies through a small qualitative study (Hjort 1975).

Sickness absence and the burdens in everyday life

Our study clearly shows that aspects of peoples' demanding and stressful work situation, as well as complicated aspects in their private situation, result in incapacities to cope with the challenges in everyday life as a whole. Previous research from a qualitative evaluation study showed that the majority of participants with long-term illnesses reported that symptoms and problems were related to their home situations and life complications (Batt-Rawden & Tellnes 2005). Illness may intrude on one's self-confidence, upsetting an already insecure balance (Bury 1982). According to Bury, patients are aware of the limits of medical knowledge; thus, it seems to be important to establish a 'body of knowledge and meaning drawn from the individual's own biography' (Bury 1982, 179). Major findings in quantitative studies show that 40–50% of sickness absence originates in working life experiences (Tellnes 1990; Tellnes et al. 1990).

The majority of the participants said that their working life had a strong impact on their sickness absence. Only a few related their sickness absence to the private sphere, and, most often, problems in their private sphere were not the only independent factors, but the determining factors. This indicates that work overload seems to be the dominant reason for sickness absence among our participants. In relation to the demand-control model (Karasek & Theorell 1990), this can be interpreted as a negative balance among strong demands, a lack of control over their own work situation, and the tasks involved. Although the participants often described their relationship to their colleagues as positive and as including social support in complicated cases, it was poor organization and leadership that seemed to reduce their energy levels and thus damage their health. There is a need to find a liveable relationship with the body – to create an acceptable bodily awareness. Achieving this may include a complex process of re-thinking, re-calling, and re-cognising life events (Van Manen 2003).

Our study supports previous findings highlighting how a complicated work and life situation decreases individuals' health. Expressions like 'burn-out', 'the last straw', 'batteries had gone flat', 'deflated', or 'hit the wall' were common among the majority of these participants (Batt-Rawden & Tellnes 2005). In this sense, illness is a disruption not only of structures of explanation and meaning for these participants, but also of the maintenance of normal relationships and the mobilisation of resources. Withdrawal from social relationships and growing social isolation are the major features of illness monitoring, and, in line with Antonovsky (1987), finding a sense of coherence in everyday life may increase self-knowledge and awareness, helping one to progress on the path to recovery.

The ability to carry out work, to engage in personal activities, and to sustain social relationships is often sufficient for people to feel that they are not ill (Anderson & Bury 1988). Health, in this sociological conceptualisation, is not a pre-given or immutable state. It is, rather, socially and active produced, performed, or negotiated as a feature of ordinary people in their everyday life. It may be difficult to be accepted or even respected when individuals have been diagnosed with problems that are not immediately apparent. For example, as one of these participants explained, 'if your foot has been casted, this is easy to spot, while stiff shoulders or mental health problems are rather more difficult to observe, perhaps even to understand'. Our participants knew and felt that the informal rules, norms, and values from their friends and relationships often influenced their daily activities. The majority hesitated to go to the local shopping centre while they were certified as sick. For the majority of the participants, this was not an option, because they expected to be interrogated and met with suspicion – to hear something like, 'Why are you here? I thought you were ill'. Some participants thought that these norms and beliefs in their social network were powerful enough to prevent people from being certified as sick, even when they really needed it. This shows that the categorization in one's social surroundings influences those on sickness absence and their identities.

Another indication of the strength of these norms is that none of the participants had been directly confronted with them during the sickness absence period. In this sense, the participants acted on the basis of suspicion, and this reveals their vulnerable situation. However, there did seem to be expectations or collective representations (Crossley 2001) from the society that enforced the participants' feelings of being 'watched' or observed, resulting in a kind of withdrawal and involuntary hibernation. Most of them were in contact with their workplace despite being certified as sick, and several visited their colleagues and patients in the nursing home. Social support from colleagues gave them strength during this difficult period of their life. Even some of those who were critical towards the leadership and the organization visited the workplace. In sum, this discussion highlights the importance of retrieving coping mechanisms, that is, a 'sense of coherence' (Antonovsky 1987), which involves how to understand, to manage and to make sense of changes in life despite being long-term certified as sick. Having a supportive social network both at home and at work will no doubt serve as a buffer against sickness absence when life becomes complicated.

Final comments

Our case study shows that employees suffering from health problems with no observable symptoms, diseases or injuries, are vulnerable to not being understood or respected in their environment. Therefore, the role of being long-term certified as sick can be difficult to handle and cope with. In this situation, the support from family and colleagues was important.

The main cause of sickness absence among employees at the nursing home was related to their working situation. During the last years, there had been increasing demands for efficiency, more demanding patients, and less control over their working situation. The consequence had been an increasing work burden on employees and, as a consequence, a high percentage of sickness absence. For the majority of the participants in our study, the solution for reducing the sickness absence seemed to be very simple and at the same time unrealistic: to provide more hands and heads to share the tasks at the nursing home. They proposed more employees so that each could have more time to provide holistic care and thus avoid having a bad conscience for not doing the right kind of work.

Without an increase in the staff, it is difficult to see how the employees could stay in their jobs permanently. One consequence could be a possible increase in sickness absence for many employees in the nursing home. In addition, for those who participated in this study, the road to recovery may take much longer than necessary. This, in turn, shows how the fragile and elderly may lack proper and sufficient care. Since there is strong pressure on the employees resulting in an increase in sickness absence, there is an evil circle, one that undermines a sense of coherence (Antonovsky 1987). We do not know if the situation at our nursing home is worse or better than the situation in other nursing homes. But many employees at the nursing home work very hard, perhaps too hard, to give the elderly patients the best care and nursing.

In this way, deficient nursing is a structural problem, and sickness absence of the employees is a symptom of this structural problem.

References

Anderson, R. & Bury, M. eds. 1988. *Living with Chronic Illness: The Experience of Patients and Their Families*. Unwin Hyman. London

Antonovsky A. 1987. *Unraveling the Mystery of Health*. San Francisco, Jossey-Bass Inc.

Antonovsky, A. 1996. 'The Salutogenetic Model as a Theory to Guide Health Promotion'. *Health Promotion International*. Vol 11, 11–16

Batt-Rawden, K. & G. Tellnes 2005. 'Nature-culture-health activities as a method of rehabilitation: an evaluation of participants' health, quality of life and function'. *International Journal of Rehabilitation Research* 28(2), 175–180

Bury, M. 1982. 'Chronic illness as biographical disruption'. *Sociology of Health and Illness* Vol 4 (2), 167–82

Crossley N. 2001. 'The phenomenological habitus and its constructions'. *Theory and Society* Vol 30/1, 81–120

Drentea P. & J. Moren-Cross 2005. 'Social Capital and Social Support on the Web: The case of an Internet Mother Site'. *Sociology of Health and Illness*, 27, 7

Eriksson, U.B. 2009. *'Man är jo inte mer än människa'. Langtidssjukskriving ur et emotionellt, rationellt och strukturellt perspektiv*. Karlstad, Karlstad University Studies No. 2

Forseth, U. 2001. *Boundless Work – Emotional Labour and Emotional Exhaustion in Interactive Service Work*. SINTEF Teknologiledelse IFIM. Dr.politavhandling. Institutt for sosiologi og statsvitenskap. Trondheim, NTNU

Gamperiene, M., A. Grimsmo, B.Å. Sørensen 2007. *Kunnskapsstatus. Tema 1: Sykefravær*. AFI-notat no. 11. Oslo, Arbeidsforskningsinstituttet

Hallsten L.& K. Isaksson 2001 'Arbetslöshet, osäker anställning och psykisk ohälsa'. I S. Marklund (ed.) *Arbetsliv och hälsa 2000*. Stockholm, Arbetarskyddstyrelsen och Arbetslivsinstitutet.

Hjort, H. 1975. 'Om å forstå det allmenne gjennom det særegne'. I Holter, H., Henriksen, H.V., Gjertsen, A. & Hjort, H. : *Familien i klassesamfunnet*. Oslo, Pax Forlag

Hochshild, A.R. 1983. *The Managed Heart. Commercialization and Human Feelings.* Berkeley and Los Angeles, University of California Press

Karasek, R. & T. Theorell 1990. *Healthy work, stress, productivity and the reconstruction of working life.* New York, Basic Books

Kruml S.M. & D. Geddes 2000. 'Exploring the dimensions of emotional labor'. *Management Communication Quarterly,* 14, 8–49

Kvale, S. 1996. *Interviews.* Thousand Oaks, CA, Sage

Maslach C. & M. Leiter 1997. *The truth about burnout.* San Fransisco, CA, Jossey-Bass

Michie, S. & S. Williams 2003. 'Reducing work related psychological ill health and sickness absence: A systematic literature review'. *Occupational and Environmental Medicine,* 60, 3–9. Socialstyrelsen 2005

Nordby, H. 2004. 'Concept possession and incorrect understanding'. *Philosophical Explorations,* 7 (1), 55–70

Olsen, K.M. 2007. 'Sykefravær – hvor mye skyldes jobben?' *Søkelys på arbeidslivet* 1, årgang 24, 53–62

Ose, S.O., H. Jensberg, R.E. Reinertsen, M. Sandsund & J.M. Dyrstad 2006. *Sykefravær. Kunnskapsstatus og problemstillinger.* Rapport. SINTEF A325. Trondheim, SINTEF

Rønning, R., K. Batt-Rawden & L.J. Solheim 2009. *Skrøpelige eldre og sjuke hjelpere.* Report ENRI 1/2009

Schabracq, M. 2003. 'What an organisation can do about its employees' well-being and health'. Schabracq, Winnubst & Cooper eds.: *The Handbook of Work and Health psychology.* 2nd edition. John Wiley & Sons

Schensul, S., Schensul, J. & LeCompte, M.D. 1999. *Wicke Essential Ethnographic Methods.* Altamira Press, London

Siegrist, J. 1996. 'Adverse health effects of high-effort/low-reward conditions'. *Journal of Occupational Health Psychology,* 1 (1), 27–41

Starrin, B. & Svensson, P.-G. eds. 1994. *Kvalitativ metod och vetenskapsteori.* Lund, Studentlitteratur

Tellnes, G. 1990. Sickness certification – an epidemiological study related to community medicine and general practice. Dissertation. University of Oslo, Department of Community Medicine, Oslo

Tellnes, G., Bruusgaard, D., Sandvik, L. 1990. 'Occupational factors in sickness certification'. *Scand J Prim Health Care,* 8, 37–44

Vahtera, J., Kiwimaki, M., et al. 2004. 'Organisational downsizing, sickness absence, and mortality: 10-town prospective cohort study'. *British Medical Journal,* 328, 555–558

Van Manen, M. 2003. *Researching Lived Experiences.* The Althouse Press, Ontario

Verhaeghe, R., Mak, R., Georges Van Maele, Marcel Kornitzer & Guy De Backer 2003. 'Job stress among middle-aged health care workers and its relation to sickness absence'. *Stress and Health* 19, 265–274 www.nav.no/243644.cms

Chapter 14

Absence and alternative learning: The Company Programme and inclusive working life as a means to reduce high school absence

Vegard Johansen, Tuva Schanke & Liv Johanne Solheim

Summary

High school absence and dropout multiplies the probability of exclusion from further education and working life, and dropouts that become employed have a higher level of sickness absence, as compared to those completing upper secondary school. Still, there are hardly any studies on school absence and young peoples' attitudes towards absence. Our chapter fills some of the gaps in our knowledge. The main aim is to evaluate to what extent a widespread European entrepreneurship program – the Company Program (CP) – changes attitudes towards absence and reduces school absence. CP is about the creation of a mini-company, and our empirical data comes from Akershus county in Norway. To create better work environments, pupils in mini-companies in Akershus County are taught about inclusive working life (IWL). A pre- and post-study indicate that CP stimulates constructive attitudes. An econometric analysis – building on a control group design – concludes that CP is able to reduce school absence.

Introduction

In February 2010, an expert group presented a series of initiatives to reduce the Norwegian sickness absence (Mykletun et al. 2010). One of their points was that dropouts, i.e. the group of young people who do not complete upper secondary school, have a higher level of sickness absence in their later employment, as compared to those who do complete upper secondary school. The expert group argued that an early focus on participation and presence could prevent sickness absence in the longer term, i.e. that school initiatives to change attitudes towards absence could reduce later work absence. The expert group concluded this section by complaining that there were far too few studies on school absence (Mykletun et al. 2010).

This chapter is an attempt to fill some of the gaps in our knowledge about school absence. We discuss the consequences and risk factors of high school absence and a policy initiative to prevent high school absence. A high level of school absence has serious consequences both in the shorter and in the longer term, and the strong correlation between absence and school dropout is particularly important (Markussen et al. 2008). Statistics Norway (2009) inform that more than three out of ten youths in Norway have not completed upper secondary school five years after they started in level 1. Dropping out of the basic education and training represents serious challenges for the individual: the probability of exclusion from further education and working life is multiplied if the basic education and training is not completed. Dropouts also represent a serious societal challenge: a recent report estimates that a reduction of the dropout rate from 30 to 20 percent for each age cohort – from 18 000 to 12 000 youths – gives an economic gain of approximately 5.4 billion NOK annually (approximately 650 million €) (Falch, Johannesen & Strøm 2009).

Even though various governments have initiated a series of education policies to reduce absence and to increase youths' propensity to stay in school, the proportion of dropouts in Norway has been the same since the 1990s. The empirical part of this chapter brings new knowledge on what to do to reduce absence and dropout. More precisely, we investigate the impact of participation in the Company Programme (CP), a widespread European entrepreneurship education programme provided by the NGO Junior Achievement

– Young Enterprise (JA-YE). JA-YE is Europe's largest provider of entrepreneurship education programmes, and CP is their premier programme. CP is a practical programme, in which children establish, run, and close a mini-company during a school year.

During the experience of running a mini-company, the children are also taught about inclusive working life (IWL). IWL is a partnership agreement between the Norwegian government, six unions, and the employer's federation.[1] It was signed in 2001 and was intended to last for four years, but it was prolonged in 2005 and in 2010 for another four years. This national programme attempted not only to tackle the problem of worker absenteeism, but also to increase the employment of functionally impaired workers and to retain ageing workers. *IWL in CP* is the name of a project running in Akershus County, and our empirical data is based on a study of this project during the years 2007–09 (Eide & Johansen 2007; Johansen & Schanke 2009). *IWL in CP* introduces the ideas of the IWL programme to pupils and uses the same methods and inclusive approach towards school absence.

Our empirical part asks two questions:
1. To what extent does participation in CP change attitudes towards school absence?
2. Are CP-participants likely to have lower school absence, as compared to other pupils?

Question 1 is answered using data from a pre- and post-test study among CP-participants in 2007. Question 2 is answered by comparing participants in CP (test group) with a group of children that did not participate in CP (control group). We used data on registered absences in 2008/09 and connected this data to answers from a questionnaire.

---

[1] The parties to the agreement are the Government, represented by the Minister of Labour and Social Inclusion, and the employer organisations NHO (Confederation of Norwegian Enterprise), HSH (Federation of Norwegian Commercial and Service Enterprises), KS (Norwegian Association of Local and Regional Authorities), NAVO (Norwegian employers' association for enterprises affiliated with the public sector), and the State as employer represented by the Minister of Government Administration and Reform, and the employee organisations LO (Norwegian Confederation of Trade Unions), Unio (Confederation of Unions for Professionals, Norway), YS (Confederation of Vocational Unions), and Akademikerne (Federation of Norwegian Professional Associations) (Ose et al. 2009).

The chapter has seven sections. The next section tells about the consequences of school absence. Section three gives details about the implementation of CP and IWL in Norway. We discuss the research design in section four. Section five presents the empirical analysis on changing attitudes to school absence and on factors influencing high school absence. Section six discusses our findings. Section seven presents some final thoughts.

The consequences of school absence

Upper secondary school is optional, yet pupils' presence or absence is registered. Schools count absence in days and hours, and they calculate absence percentages. This registration is an incentive for pupils to attend lessons, and the information provided is valued by teachers and the school administration as an important tool for helping pupils.

Tellnes (1989) identifies three types of absence from work, and these categories are also relevant when studying school absence. *Absenteeism* refers to unexcused absence (shirking, lateness, inertia, and truancy), and it is estimated that 20 percent of the total school absence is unlawful or unjustified (Ingul 2005). The lawful part of absence consists of *leave* (absence caused by civic duties, medical appointments, political work, and class representation) and *sickness absence* (absence caused by disease, injuries, or illness). If documented (e.g. certified sickness absence by a doctor or parents, documents proving class representation and political work), pupils have a right to 14 days reduction in their annual school absence.

Most children have a low level of absence, and this represents few challenges. A high level of absence, on the other hand, creates a problem that is stressful for children, families, and school personnel. Failing to attend school has significant short- and long-term effects on children's social, emotional, and educational development, and we will give some examples. We begin with the short-term effects.

Short-term consequences of high school absence

The level of absence is relevant for the certificate for upper secondary education and training. The first point is that the absence at each level is given in days and hours on the certificate. The second point is that a high level of unlawful absence could lead to lower marks for order and conduct. The third point is that a high level of absence could result in failure to pass upper secondary school and not get a certificate. If the pupil cannot document his competence in a subject (non-participation at tests and assignments), the teacher is in no position to make an academic judgment (Ministry of education and research 1998). According to Statistics Norway (2009), eight percent of those starting in 2003 were still registered in upper secondary school in 2008 due to the failure to pass one or more subjects. A fourth point is that a high level of absence might negatively affect the average mark. There are, of course, many factors that affect marks (abilities, interest in the subject, teaching methods, peers, parents, and many others), and absence could be one negative factor. If a pupil is not present, he or she might miss the explanation of crucial material, or miss homework and assignments, or fall behind and have a hard time catching up with the rest of the class. Oral presentation is also an important part of the evaluation in many subjects.

In addition to these 'certificate-consequences', high school absence can have a negative effect on work applications. School absence is of no significance when applying for higher education, but it does matter to employers when hiring students part-time and offering apprenticeships. A longitudinal study of more than 9 000 schoolchildren showed that good marks and low absence was the most important criteria when employers allocated apprenticeships (Markussen et al. 2008).

A high level of school absence is not only correlated with academic challenges and problems getting work or an apprenticeship; it is also a marker for social or mental problems. Kearney (2001) explains that school absence can spread to other social arenas, and the longer a pupil has been absent, the harder it is to help or treat him or her. A related point is the strong correlation between a high level of school absence and dropout, and with this, an increased probability of exclusion from further education and working life as a young adult. The next section deals with dropout and marginalization.

Long-term consequences of dropout

The school is an important arena for socialising young people into society both as citizens and as participants in the labour market. In the past decades, the length of the basic education and training has been prolonged, and there are an increasing number of possibilities in higher education. For the majority, basic education and training is expected to be the start of further education to attain the competence necessary to go into different professional positions in society.

Young people who do not live up to the expectation of completing upper secondary school are in danger of being marginalized and even excluded from important arenas in society later in their lives. School absence may be a first step towards dropout from school, and this may put them in a difficult position when they try to enter further education and find a job in a society in which most jobs require formal competence. There are variations among local labour markets: in some places, there are industry and service jobs, which recruit young people with only basic education and training (Heggen, Jørgensen & Paulgaard 2002). Still, it was recently estimated that, in 2025, there will be demand for more than basic education and training in 97 percent of the labour market (Government White Paper 44 2008–09). It is obvious that high school absence followed by dropout can exclude young people from the labour market and put them in a marginalized position.

To be in a marginalized position impedes the possibility to move either towards exclusion or towards inclusion (Svedberg 1995). Pupils who have dropped out of upper secondary school have the possibility to return to school and complete their education later or to find jobs that do not require upper secondary education. Expected income is considerably lower among dropouts, as compared to youths with basic education and training (Opheim 2009). For some, dropout is a step towards exclusion from the labour market. In the last few years, there has been a significant increase among young people on disability pension (Solheim 2010). People on disability pension are usually excluded from the labour market, and very few return to the labour market after a period on disability pension, even if there are initiatives to stimulate a return to labour market. According to a study of all Norwegian citizens born between 1967 and 1976, educational attainment is the single most important variable when predicting disability pension. The chance for disability pension is five times higher among those who did not complete basic education by the age of 20, as compared to those who did complete it (Gravseth 2009).

Participation in the labour market has an important influence on people's economic situation both during working age and during retirement. Low or no income means low pension, and people in low-income jobs often have less control over their job situation and more physically strenuous work. Educational attainment is also a key factor for health and social functioning:

People with low educational attainment have more health problems, as compared to those with higher education (Elstad 2000), they are overrepresented among receivers of social benefits (van der Wel et al. 2006), and their suicide rates are twice as high (Gravseth 2009). This gives an indication of the vulnerability experienced by some of the young people in basic education and training – representing a special challenge for both the school and society.

The Company Programme and inclusive working life

Over the past decade, various initiatives have been put forth to reduce school absence and dropout rates. Strengthening career guidance in lower secondary school is important in order to reduce the large share of pupils choosing the 'wrong' education programme, a good system for registration of absence is important for quick follow-ups of pupils with social and academic challenges, and many schools choose to run special programmes for exposed groups (like pupils living by themselves in a rented room or small apartment) (Buland & Havn 2007). Our chapter investigates schools using the Company programme (CP) as a pedagogical alternative generally and particularly for pupils with difficulties in the traditional and ordinary education. CP is offered in 40 countries and considered a 'Best Practice entrepreneurship education programme' (European Commission 2005).

Traditionally schools' gave little attention to entrepreneurship education. Due to a 'new' emphasis on entrepreneurship in European and Norwegian education systems, more and more children and youths take part in entrepreneurship courses (Johansen, Schanke & Hauge 2009). Junior Achievement – Young Enterprise (JA-YE) offers 'learning by doing' programmes for all stages of education from kindergarten to higher education. The Norwegian branch is financially supported by the ministries of Education and Research, of Business and Industry, and of Local Government and Regional Development (Junior Achievement-Young Enterprise Norway 2009).

CP reaches approximately ten percent of all children in Norwegian upper secondary school. CP gives young people the opportunity to prepare for working life through the experience of running their own company, supported by volunteer advisers from business and by their teacher. In a school year, the pupils sell stock, elect officers, produce and market products or services, keep records, conduct stockholders' meetings, and liquidate. The programme provides a real experience of business enterprise, and the mini-companies participate in National and European Competitions and Trade Fairs (Junior Achievement-Young Enterprise Norway 2009). CP prepares young people for the real world by showing them how to generate wealth and to manage it, how to create jobs which make their communities more robust, and how to apply entrepreneurial thinking to the workplace. The objectives of CP are to raise young people's awareness of self-employment as a career option, as well as to promote personal qualities relevant to entrepreneurship and other aspects of life (creativity, cooperation abilities, problem-solving abilities, and spirit of initiative) (Johansen, Schanke & Hauge 2009).

To create better work environments, pupils in mini-companies in Akershus County are taught about inclusive working life (IWL). IWL is a partnership agreement between the Norwegian government, six unions, and the employer's federation. IWL is about creating a work environment that prevents sickness absence and expulsion and increases the focus on job presence. All public and private enterprises are invited to sign an IWL agreement, to make their own local goals to reduce sickness absence, and to include vulnerable groups. In 2009, 56 percent of all Norwegian employees worked in an IWL enterprise (Solheim 2010). The evaluation of the IWL agreement showed that it was insufficient to reduce average sickness absence, but one positive finding was that many enterprises had improved follow-up practices with respect to people with long-term sickness absence (Ose et al. 2009).

Using the national IWL agreement as a starting point, the project *IWL in CP* was launched in 2006. Pupils learn about IWL in courses and school visits by Akershus Labour and Welfare Service, JA-YE Akershus created a guide on IWL with both practical and theoretical assignments, and all mini-companies compete to be the best IWL-company in the county. To take part in the IWL-project, all pupils in a mini-company must sign the IWL-agreement (similar to the 'real' version), and they commit themselves to prevent absence and social exclusion, not only in the mini-company but also at their school. The latter objective is the focus of part 5 in this chapter, in which we evaluate to what extent *IWL in CP* changes attitudes towards absence and reduces absence.

Research design

In investigating the effects of education programmes, we aim at answering this question: what would have happened with the participants, if they had not participated in the programme? Considering CP, we are able to observe the factual situation (what happens to CP-participants), but it is not possible to observe the counterfactual situation (what would have happened to participants had they not been included in CP). Hence, it is necessary to approximate the counterfactual situation.

Most evaluation studies rely on comparison-group designs when approximating the counterfactual situation (Mohr 1995). In such designs, a group of participants (the test group) are compared to a group of non-participants (the control group), where the latter group is used as an estimate of the counterfactual situation. The difference in the average score (on some indicator) between these two groups is then used as the estimate of the causal influence of the programme. Most evaluation research is done using quasi-experimental designs, in which the allocation of individuals to either the test or control-group is non-random. This is unfortunate, since non-randomness creates several statistical problems associated with unobserved heterogeneity, self-selection, and selection bias.[2] Therefore, random assignment of individuals to the test and control group is judged as the 'gold standard' within the evaluation literature (Mohr 1995).

Part 5.2 is a study of school absence in which a group of 17- to 19-year-olds who participated in CP are compared to a group of non-participants. The children themselves do not influence the decision to participate in CP or not, and, in theory, the children could have been randomly assigned into either CP-participation or non-participation. In practice, the random assignment rule is violated. One point is that the school leadership decides whether or not their school should participate in CP, and CP is more common among vocational education programmes. To control for the possible

---

[2] The main problem is the possible existence of a correlation between the factors that influence assignment outcome in either the test or control group and the dependent variable. If one is not able to control for all the factors that are both correlated with assignment outcome and the dependent variable using for instance regression analysis, the estimate of the influence of the programme will be biased in quasi-experimental research designs (Mohr 1995).

overrepresentation of schoolchildren in vocational programmes in the CP-group, we include a dummy variable on 'education programme' in our analysis (see part 5.2). Another point of note is that most schools in the sample systematically allocated children with difficulties in traditional and ordinary education to take part in CP. It is argued that these children should take part in CP in the hopes that they might benefit from a more practical and less academic learning environment. We cannot control for the selection of children who are likely to have a high level of absence to the CP-group, and it challenges the 'true experimental nature' of our design. We are, however, able to control for a dozen other independent variables potentially affecting school absence (see part 5.2)

Our study also concerns attitudes to absence and inclusive working life. In this study, a single sample of CP-participants were asked a series of questions before and after CP-participation, and the McNemar test is used to evaluate whether *IWL in CP* had an impact. It is worth noting that comparisons of pre-test and post-test results may be inaccurate because participants may have limited knowledge at the beginning of a programme that prevents them from accurately assessing baseline attitudes. In this case, when asked before *IWL in CP*, schoolchildren might have had problems answering about their attitudes if we used terms they would only learn about in the project (e.g., inclusive working life, job presence). To solve this problem, we asked about absence in a more straightforward way that children could reasonably answer both before and after CP-participation.

IWL in CP and school absence

This part presents the empirical analysis. The first piece is our analysis of attitudes towards absence. The second piece concerns factors explaining school absence.

Attitudes towards absence

The empirical data on attitudes is based on responses from 120 CP-participants who completed our web-based questionnaires in January (pre-test) and May 2007 (post-test) (Eide & Johansen 2007). The response rate was acceptable (47). Even though 120 respondents is a rather small sample, we hope to find some indications if *IWL in CP* changes attitudes towards absence.

The respondents were asked to assess a longer series of assertions/questions about absence, and we present four of these in table 1. To simplify, results are recoded from five to two alternatives: agree and disagree/uncertain. Data is analysed using McNemar's test, a non-parametric method used on 2×2-tables. This test presents p-values, which measures how probable it is that there was no change in attitudes before (pre) and after (post) participation in CP. If p-values are low (p< 0.1), then the effects are statistical significant, i.e. that there probably was a change in attitudes.

Table 1: Changing attitudes towards absence, percent and p-value.

Claims/questions	Pre-test			Post-test			
	A	DU	Sum	A	DU	Sum	p
My absence is also other peoples' concern	37	63	100	56	44	100	***
A high level of absence is a marker of discomfort	25	75	100	36	64	100	*
Absence does matter even if the work is done	33	67	100	39	61	100	
Did you expect/did you experience reduced absence	54	46	100	33	67	100	***

N = 120, *** Significant at 0.01, ** Significant at 0.05, * Significant at 0.1.
A = Agree, D = Disagree, U = Uncertain, p = p-value

Table 1 tells us that CP matters. After participation, a larger share of respondents consider that their absence affects other people, that a high level of absence is a marker of discomfort, and that job presence is important even if the work is done. More precisely:
- More respondents consider that their 'absence is a concern for other people' after participation (56 percent) than before (37 percent). This shift is significant.
- More respondents consider that 'a high level of absence is a marker of discomfort' after participation (36 percent) than before (25 percent). This shift is significant.
- A somewhat higher share of respondents considers that 'job presence is important even if the work is done' after participation (39 percent) than before (33 percent).

- 54 percent of the respondents expected that the project would reduce their own and classmates' school absence, and 33 percent experienced that it did.

Factors explaining school absence

The surveys in 2007 dealt with attitudes, while our research in 2008/2009 looked into the actual absence. In the latter study, questionnaires were answered in writing at school. Using a 'key' (pupils' school-number), we were able to connect answers from a questionnaire with the registered absences that school year (Johansen & Schanke 2009). Six schools and twelve classes participated in this part of the project. Through an extensive process, we managed to recruit 272 of 282 respondents to give us access to their registered absence, a response rate of more than 90 percent. About 40 percent of the respondents were CP-participants (test group), and 60 percent were non-participants (control group). Even if we are satisfied with the response rate, it is worth noting that we are dealing with a rather small sample (272 respondents), and results should be interpreted cautiously.

Table 2: Shares of respondents with low absence (0–4.9 percent), medium absence (5–9.9 percent) and high absence (10 percent or more), percent.

Groups	Percent
Low absence (0–4.9)	50
Medium absence (5–9.9)	32
High absence (10+)	18
Sum	100

N = 272

Reducing the share of pupils with a high level of school absence is considered a key performance criterion of *IWL in CP*. Even though there is no general rule, many schools use 10 percent absence as a norm for what they refer to as 'high absence'.[3] Table 2 shows that half of the respondents' have a low level of

---

[3] The documentation report (Johansen & Schanke 2009) argues in favour of calculating absence percentages. One reason to calculate absence percentages is to have a single measure (and not two: days and hours). Another reason is that schools are concerned with overall absence percentages and calculate such measures themselves. A third reason for using absence percentages is that vocational education programmes and the programme for specialization in general studies have different hours in a school year, the former 1330

absence (50 percent), one in three have a medium level (32 percent), and one in six (18 percent) have a high level of absence. In the remainder of this section, we explore the division between pupils with high absence (10+ percent) and low/medium absence (0–9.9 percent).

Regression analysis is an attempt to understand how a set of independent variables (explanatory variables) affects a particular dependent variable. In our case, *school absence* is the dependent variable. School absence has two values: 0 (low/medium absence) and 1 (high absence). Logistic regression is suitable when the dependent variable has two values (Hamilton 1992).

The main point of our analysis is to determine whether or not CP-participants are less likely to have a high level of absence than other pupils. Our survey includes questions on a range of background variables that will enable us to control for a range of 'competing explanations' in our assessment of the impact of CP on high absence. Figure 1 presents the explanatory model of variations in absence.

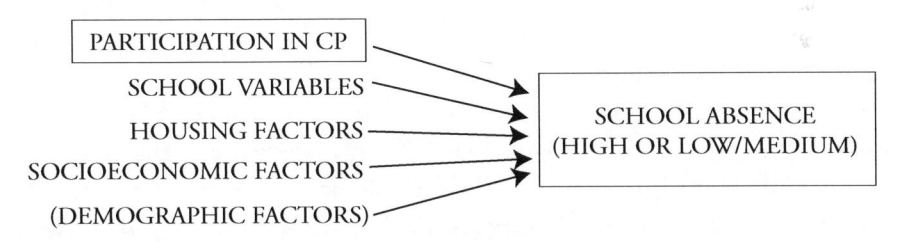

Figure 1: Variables explaining level of absence (high and low/medium).

The main explanatory dimension is CP-participation. On the one hand, CP-participants are taught about IWL and commit themselves to prevent school absence. They are, thus, expected to have a lower level of absence compared to non-participants. On the other hand, the CP-group consists of a large share of pupils having difficulties in traditional education and are likely to have a high level of absence. The chosen variable – Participation in CP – is a dummy variable with two values: CP-participation equals 0 (reference category) and non-participation equals 1.

The first set of control variables are school variables: educational programme and level. The programme for specialization in general studies has a

---

hours and the latter 1140 hours. To make a valid comparison of pupils from different programmes, we have to calculate absence percentages.

lower dropout rate, as compared to vocational programmes (Markussen et al. 2008). It is, thus, expected that vocational programmes will have a relatively high rate of absence. Our model compares vocational programmes (value 1) with general studies (value 0). We also expect pupils in upper secondary level 3 to have a higher level of absence, as compared to those in levels 1 and 2. There are many circumstances in level 3 supporting this expectation, like driving lessons and parties and festivities ('russetid'). Our model compares level 3 (value 1) and levels 1 and 2 (value 0).

The second set of control variables are housing factors: travel time and renting or living at home. Travel time refers to the number of minutes the pupil uses to get from his home to school, and it is suggested that long travel time increases the probability of a high level of absence (Buland & Havn 2007). Our model compares pupils with 1 hour or more total travel time from home to school and back (value 1) and those using 0–59 minutes (value 0). Former studies show that pupils living by themselves in a rented room or small apartment are particularly exposed to high absence (Wiborg & Rønning 2005). Our model compares pupils renting a room (value 1) and those living at home (value 0).

The third set of control variables are socioeconomic factors. Many studies indicate that parents' participation in the labour market and parents' educational attainment are determinants for academic skills and dropout. We expect that those with two working parents have the lowest levels of absence. Our model compares pupils with two working parents (value 0) and those with neither or only one parent working (value 1). Due to lack of explanatory power, the final model does not include the education variable (see table 4).

The final control variables are demographic factors: gender and ethnic origin. Both variables are excluded in the final analysis due to lack of explanatory power (see table 4).

The first column in table 3 tells the name of the variables included in the analysis. The second column shows the unstandardized Coefficient (B): the average increase in the dependent variable with one measurement increase in X (independent variable) when other independent variables are held constant. The third column presents the standard of errors (SE), a measure of sample-to-sample variation (Hamilton 1992). We will focus our comments on p-values (p), the odds ratio (Exp(B)) and Nagelkerke R^2.

Table 3: The factors explaining high school absence, unstandardized coefficients (B), p-value (p), standard error (SE) and odds ratio (Exp(B)).

Variables	B	P	SE	Exp(B)
Constant	-4.86	***	1.12	0.01
Non-CP-participation	0.66		0.45	1.93
Vocational programme	1.47	***	0.45	4.36
Level 3	1.08	*	0.66	2.93
Long travel time	0.66	*	0.36	1.94
Renting an apartment/room	1.77	***	0.68	5.84
One parent or zero parents working	1.00	**	0.43	2.72
Nagelkerke R²	0.15			

*** Significant at 0.01, ** Significant at 0.05, * Significant at 0.1.
Reference categories: CP-participation; general studies; levels 1&2; short travel time; living at home; two parents working

R^2 is a measure of goodness-of-fit used in linear regression models. Corresponding, logistic regression models enable calculations of R^2-like measures, and the most reported is Nagelkerke R^2. Nagelkerke R^2 ranges from 0 to 1, and higher values indicate better model fit. Nagelkerke R^2 is 0.15, and there are six independent variables in our model. Our interpretation is that the model includes many important variables, but most of the variation in school absence is unexplained.

P-values represent a second way to analyze the impact of different variables (see also section 5.1). There are statistical differences (p<0.05) on high absence for: vocational versus general studies, renting a room versus living at home, and two parents working versus one/zero parents working. The model also indicates that level, travel time, and CP-participation matters, even if p-values are higher than 0.05.

Odds ratios (Exp(B)) represent the third way to analyze the impact of variables. When the odds ratio is close to 1, we do not have any particular effect; the higher it is over 1, the stronger the positive effect, and the closer it is to 0, the stronger the negative effect. The impact of participation in CP is as follows: non-participants in CP are 1.9 times more likely to have high school absence compared to CP-participants. The most important variable is education programme, and those in vocational programmes are 4.4 times more likely to have high absence compared to pupils in the general studies. Another key variable is housing, and the odds ratio of high school absence among schoolchildren renting an apartment/room is 5.8 contrasted to those living at home.

Discussion of the results

There is a close relationship between changes in society and changes in the educational system. Over the past decades, changes in the labour market have interacted with an increasing education level in the population. In this way, education is not only an entrance into the labour market, but also an important contributor to the transformation of working life and of the standard of living (Hernes 2010). The most important change in the labour market is, perhaps, the dramatic decline of unskilled workers, and the increasing demand for education. Young people who do not live up to the expectations to qualify for the modern labour market, are, thus, vulnerable to marginalization and social exclusion. This is not a preferred position for the individual. For society, a reduction of dropouts will be a considerable gain (Falch, Johannesen & Strøm 2009).

In the 1990s, basic education and training was extended to last 13 years (6–19 years of age). An important goal of the school reforms in 1994 and 1997 was to the meet the demand from the labour market regarding more competence. Among the goals of reform 94 was that everybody should have a enough 'general studies' to make them eligible for higher education later on, which in practice meant more theory in vocational studies. Perhaps vocational studies became too theoretical: compared to 18 percent of pupils in the general studies, 45 percent in vocational programmes had not completed upper secondary school five years after they started in level 1 (Statistics Norway 2009).

In the past decades, a series of education policy initiatives has been introduced to reduce high school absence and dropout (Buland & Havn 2007). We decided to evaluate the impact of a particular project called *IWL in CP*, i.e. Inclusive Working Life in the Company Programme. Former studies on CP have shown its advantages as a pedagogical alternative for pupils with difficulties in traditional and ordinary education (Johansen, Schanke & Hauge 2009), but we did not know whether it would change attitudes towards absence and reduce the actual school absence.

The first part of the empirical analysis was a pre-test and a post-test among 120 CP-participants on their attitudes towards absence. Our results indicated changing attitudes: after CP-participation, a larger share of respondents consider that their absence affects other people, that a high level of absence is a marker of discomfort, and that job presence is important even if the work is done. These results give some support to the idea that CP changes attitudes and, thus, could decrease school absence and dropout.

The second part was an analysis on the actual school absence among 272 pupils: 40 percent participated in CP (test group) and 60 percent did not (control group). The indicator used was high school absence – referring to an absence percentage of ten or more. 18 percent of the respondents belonged to this group. Our model indicated that CP could reduce the percentage of pupils with a high level of school absence: non-participants in CP are 1.9 times more likely than CP-participants to have high school absence. Even if the CP-group consisted of many children with difficulties in traditional education and who were likely to have a high level of absence, the share of high absence in the test group (CP) was lower than that in the control group (non-CP). In addition to selection of education programme and possible participation in CP, the analysis also indicated correlations between other independent variables and high school absence. There are three risk groups for high school absence: pupils renting an apartment or room, pupils with long travel time, and pupils with zero or one working parent. More research is needed in order to find appropriate initiatives to prevent the marginalisation of these groups.

Considering that absence correlates with dropout, there could be high economic rewards for implementing projects such as *IWL in CP* in schools. According to the analysis, CP is considerably more important for high school absence, as compared to variables like gender, ethnic background, and parents' educational attainment. Thus, our econometric analysis suggests that CP can stimulate children with different social backgrounds to stay at school.

Final comments

Dropout from basic education and training represents serious challenges for the individual and for society. The probability of exclusion from further education and working life is multiplied if the basic education and training is not completed, and dropouts also have a higher level of sickness absence if they become employed when compared to those completing upper secondary school. Identifying risk factors for high school absence and dropout is necessary to choose the correct policies to reduce these problems. It is a paradox that the proportion of dropouts has been the same since the 1990s, in spite of various attempts to increase youths' inclination to stay in school (Statistics Norway 2009). Our study might bring new knowledge on what to do. Even if the samples in our surveys are small (120 and 272 pupils respectively), even if the study is done in one particular county with its particular geography and context (Akershus), and even if we have not controlled for all variables relevant to absence, our results are pretty convincing that the implementation of projects such as *IWL in CP* can stimulate attitudes and reduce absence. And it is not only this particular study, but a series of studies on CP conducted over the past five years that indicate the positive effects of CP (Johansen, Schanke & Hauge 2009). These studies tell us that many pupils, in particular those experiencing low levels of mastery in the traditional subjects, can get a boost when they participate in CP, where practical and theoretical learning work together.

References

Buland, Trond & Vidar Havn 2007. *Intet menneske er en øy: Rapport fra evalueringen av tiltak i Satsing mot frafall.* Trondheim, SINTEF (SINTEF report no. A07023)

Eide, Trude Hella & Vegard Johansen 2007. *Jakten på arbeidsgleden i ungdomsbedriften. Resultater fra følgeevaluering av prosjektet.* Lillehammer, Eastern Norway Research Institute (ENRI-report 09/2007)

European Commission 2005. *Triggering a new generation of entrepreneurs: students breathe new life into EU-entrepreneurship.* Brussels, European Commission

Elstad, Jon Ivar 2000. *Social inequalities in health and their explanations.* Oslo, Norwegian Social Research (NSC-report 09/2000)

Falch, Torberg, Anne Borge Johannesen & Bjarne Strøm 2009. *Kostnader av frafall i videregående opplæring.* Trondheim, Centre for Economic Research at NTNU (CER-report 08/2009)

Gravseth, Hans Magne 2009. *Disability and suicide in early adulthood in a life course perspective - A register-based cohort study of Norwegians born 1967–1976.* Oslo, University of Oslo (Series of dissertations at Faculty of Medicine no. 775)

Government White Paper no. 44 (2008–2009) *Utdanningslinja.* Oslo, Norwegian Parliament

Hamilton, Lawrence 1992. *Regression with graphics: A second course in applied statistics.* California, Wadsworth Inc

Heggen, Kåre, Gunnar Jørgensen & Gry Paulgaard 2005. *De andre. Ungdom, risikosoner og marginalisering.* Bergen, Fagbokforlaget

Hernes, Gudmund 2010. *Gull av gråstein. Tiltak for å redusere frafall i videregående opplæring.* Oslo, Fafo Institute for Labour and Social Research (FAFO-report 03/2010)

Ingul, Jon Magne 2005. 'Skolevegring hos barn og ungdom'. Voksne for barn: *Se meg!,* 27–39

Johansen, Vegard & Tuva Schanke 2009. *Trivsel og fravær i videregående opplæring.* Lillehammer, Eastern Norway Research Institute (ENRI-report 08/2009)

Johansen, Vegard, Tuva Schanke & Atle Hauge 2009. 'Den skal tidlig krøkes -entreprenørskap i skolen'. Johnstad, Tom & Atle Hauge eds.: *Innovasjon og samhandling - aktører, systemer og initiativ i Innlandet,* 189–210

Johnstad, Tom & Atle Hauge eds. 2009. *Innovasjon og samhandling - aktører, systemer og initiativ i Innlandet.* Stange, Oplandske forlag.

Junior Achievement-Young Enterprise Norway 2009. Årsrapport Ungt Entreprenørskap. Oslo, Ungt Entreprenørskap

Kearney, Christopher 2001. *School refusal behavior in youth: a functional approach to assessment and treatment.* Washington DC, American Psychological Association

Markussen, Eifrid et al. 2008. *Bortvalg og kompetanse.* Oslo, Norwegian Institute for Studies in Innovation, Research and Education (NIFU STEP-report 13/2008)

Ministry of education & research 1998. *Lov om grunnskolen og den vidaregåande opplæringa (opplæringslova).* Oslo, Ministry of education & research

Mohr Lawrence 1995. *Impact analysis for programme evaluation.* London, Sage Publications

Opheim, Vibeke 2009. 'Kostnader ved frafall: Hva betyr frafall i videregående opplæring for inntekt blant ulike grupper yrkesaktiv ungdom?' *Søkelys på arbeidslivet* no. 3, 325–40

Mykletun, Arnstein et al. 2009. *Tiltak for reduksjon i sykefravær: Aktiviserings- og nærværsreform.* Oslo, Ministry of Labour

Ose, Solveig et al. 2009. *Evaluering av IA-avtalen (2001–2009).* Trondheim, SINTEF (SINTEF report no. A11960)

Solheim, Liv Johanne 2010. 'Inclusive working life and value conflict in Norway'. *International Journal of Sociology and Social Policy,* no. 7/8, 399–411.

Statistics Norway 2009 [cit. 30.06.2010]. *Utdanning.* <http://www.ssb.no/utdanning_tema>

Svedberg, Lars 1995. *Marginalitet.* Lund, Studentlitteratur

Tellnes, Gunnar 1989. 'Sickness certification in general practice: a review'. *Family Practice* no. 1, 58–65

Wiborg, Agnete & Wenche Rønning 2005. *Frafall, bortvalg, avbrudd eller skoleslutt? Frafall innen videregående skole i Nordland i skoleåret 2004–2005.* Bodø, Nordland Research Institute (NRI-memo 1013)

Van der Wel, Kjetil ed. 2006. *Funksjonsevne blant langtidsmottakere av sosialhjelp.* Oslo, Oslo University college

Voksne for barn 2005. *Se meg!* Oslo, Voksne for barn

Appendix

Table 4: Original model of the factors explaining high school absence.

Variables	B		SE	Exp(B)
Constant	-3.49	***	0.87	0.03
Non-participation in CP	0.69		0.46	1.99
Vocational programme	1.50	***	0.46	4.48
Level 3	1.09	*	0.66	2.97
Long travel time	0.68	*	0.36	1.97
Renting apartment/room	1.76	***	0.68	5.81
One parent or zero parents' working	1.05	**	0.47	2.85
Parent(s) with high education	0.07		0.38	1.08
Girl	0.12		0.37	1.12
Norwegian	0.07		0.50	1.07
Nagelkerke R2	0.15			

*** Significant at 0.01, ** Significant at 0.05, * Significant at 0.1.
Reference categories: CP-participation; general studies; levels 1&2; short travel time; living at home; two parents' working; two parent(s) with low education; boy; immigrant background

Chapter 15

Social factors and long-term sickness absence: The need for a broader approach

Vegard Johansen & Rolf Rønning

Summary

Variations in sickness absence at the individual level are often explained by demographic factors (e.g., gender, age), family relations (e.g., household type), socio-economic status (e.g., education) and workplace characteristics (e.g., psycho-social). Our econometric analysis of long-term sickness absence (LTSA), defined as the sum of 28 or more absentee days within the prior year, indicates that life-style and social capital also matter. Indicators of a poor life-style, such as daily smoking and obesity, are connected to higher levels of LTSA. Indicators of social integration in the community also correlate with LTSA: respondents hardly ever visited by friends, family, and neighbours and who lack a friend to confide in are overrepresented with LTSA. Our findings indicate that it may be useful to conduct more research on the connections between indicators of social capital, life-style and sickness absence. The data used is from a quantitative level of living study conducted in two 'typical' Norwegian municipalities, Dovre and Lesja.

Introduction

The level of sickness absence is a serious challenge in Norway. In the last decade, the mean rate of doctor-certified sickness absence in Norway was more than six percent. The mean increased to more than seven percent when self-certified absence was included (Statistics Norway 2010). Furthermore, there was an increase in sickness absence in the latter part of this time period, most notably in 2009. At the same time, the distribution of sickness absence is skewed, and a small group of workers account for most of the total sickness absence. In 2008, approximately twelve percent of the workforce accounted for 80 percent of the doctor-certified sickness absence in Norway (Mykletun et al. 2009).

Some groups of workers are more vulnerable to sickness absence than others. Differences in levels of sickness absence are understood and explained by demographic factors (e.g., gender, age), socio-economic status (e.g., type of work, education) and workplace characteristics (e.g., physical and psychosocial) (Ose et al. 2006; Lidwall 2010). The purpose of this empirically-oriented chapter is to discuss how social factors influence sickness absence. We shall restrict our analysis to long-term sickness absence (LTSA), here defined as the sum of 28 or more absentee days within the prior year. We focus on LTSA for two reasons. The first reason is that short-term sickness absence (STSA) does not require sickness certification from a doctor, and STSA is often used to respond to common and minor problems. The second is that those with LTSA account for most of the total sickness absence, and if we are to reduce the total level of sickness absence in our society, groups vulnerable for LTSA must be the target group (Mykletun et al. 2009).

The data used to investigate how social factors influence LTSA comes from a quantitative level-of-living study conducted in two Norwegian municipalities, Dovre and Lesja (Johansen & Rønning 2009). Dovre and Lesja are representatives of 'the typical Norwegian municipality' with regard to both level of sickness absence and size. First, compared to the national average, the doctor-certified sickness absence in Dovre and Lesja was just below the national level (Statistics Norway 2010). Second, more than half of Norway's 430 municipalities have less than 5 000 inhabitants, and both Lesja (2 000 inhabitants) and Dovre (3 000 inhabitants) belong to this category.

Factors of relevance to long-term sickness absence are investigated by different professions using various theories, methods, and approaches (Palmer 2004; Ose et al. 2006; Gamperiene et al. 2007). The models applied most frequently seem to include three elements: individual factors, aspects of work, and aspects of society (Lidwall 2010). We have chosen to focus on individual factors and psycho-social working conditions. Aspects of society (e.g. unemployment levels) and other work aspects (e.g. physical working conditions) are not accounted for. Still our survey data includes questions on a range of dimensions and allows for rather complex modelling. The data enables us to control for 'competing' influences on self-reported LTSA. The relevant dimensions looked into are: demography, education, sector, psycho-social working conditions, social capital, and life-style. Since our data consists of self-reported information, our article is a supplement to analyses based on official registers that only covers doctor-certified sickness absence.

The chapter has six sections. The next section presents our theoretical considerations and choice of variables. The third section presents our data, and section four gives a descriptive analysis of sickness absence in Dovre and Lesja. The fifth section presents the empirical analysis of factors influencing LTSA. The final section discusses main findings and what we can learn from these results.

Theoretical reflections and choice of variables

This section presents theoretical considerations and choices of variables. The phenomenon investigated is long-term sickness absence (LTSA), and we will explore its relations with: a) demography, education, and sector, b) psycho-social working conditions, c) social capital, and d) life-style. In all, we present 15 variables expected to be relevant to self-reported LTSA. The effects of these variables will later on be analyzed using logistic regression.

Long-term sickness absence (LTSA)

The assessment of sickness absence in general – and LTSA in particular – is a challenge. There are three points to be made: first, sickness absence is not the only type of absence from work; second, there is an array of ways to measures sickness absence; and third, the literature on LTSA refers to various cut-off points (in number of days) for what counts as long-term sickness absence.

In his important review of the practice of sickness certification in general, Tellnes (1989a) identifies three types of absence from work. *Absenteeism* refers to unexcused absence (e.g., shirking, lateness), *leave* refers to when a person is allowed to be absent from work (e.g., civic duties, children's sickness, medical appointments), and *sickness absence* is most frequently used when absence from work is caused by disease, injuries, or illness. Sickness absence includes both sickness certification by a doctor and self-certification, i.e. a person's own declaration of sickness as a cause for absence.

Tellnes (1989) goes on to evaluate eleven measures used in the literature on sickness certification in general practice. He separates these measures in two major groups: rates and duration. Hensing (2009) uses the same division in her recent article on the application of five basic ways of assessing sickness absence in epidemiologic studies. *Frequency* refers to sickness absence episodes, *incidence rate* refers to estimates of frequency per person-time, *duration of absence* refers to mean/median days spent away during each episode of sickness absence, *length* is often measured as the number of days of sickness absence, and *cumulative incidence* is used to assess the proportion of individuals absent during a specified time period. Our data reflects *cumulative incidence* in a discussion about the proportion of individuals in Dovre and Lesja being absent due to sickness in the previous twelve months. This is useful for an assessment of the burden of sickness absence in these municipalities. *Length* is reflected in the distribution of absent days per worker in Dovre and Lesja. Studies of *length* are often limited to analyzing sickness absence of certain duration (Hensing 2009), and we will focus on those with LTSA. LTSA refers to situations in which people are incapable of work for several weeks.

In his thesis, Lidwall (2010) presents a literature overview of definitions of LTSA and how LTSA is measured empirically. Lidwall shows the huge variation in cut-off points for LTSA, such as three days (a Finnish study), seven days (a British study), 28 days (various Swedish and Norwegian studies), 56 days (various Danish and Norwegian studies), 60 and 90 days (various Swedish studies). This tells us that LTSA is a phenomenon defined very differently, and the choice of cut-off point is rather arbitrary and depends on the availability of data. The divergent cut-off points obviously pose a problem when trying to compare results of different studies: it is unreasonable to match up studies referring to LTSA as three days and those referring to LTSA as 90 days.

We choose to divide between respondents with less and more than 28 days of sickness absence in the previous twelve months. Defining LTSA as at least 28 days within the last year, we use a common cut-off point in LTSA research. This cut-off point excludes respondents with frequent short-term sickness absence (e.g., patterns of absence due to minor illnesses) and includes those with doctor-certified absence and a combination of doctor-certified and self-certified absence. Our dependent variable has the value of 0 (no sickness absence or short-term sickness absence) or 1 (long-term sickness absence).

Demographic factors, education and sector

Gender and *age* are important demographic factors. In Norway and other countries, it is a well known that women run a higher risk of LTSA than men (Palmer 2004; Ose et al. 2006; Gamperiene et al. 2007; Statistics Norway 2010). Several hypotheses have been put forward to explain gender differences with regard to LTSA, such as women's reproductive role, women's responsibilities for the family, and the fact that men and women have different working conditions (Palmer 2004; Dyrstad et al. 2005). In the regression model, men equal 0 (reference category), and women equal 1.

Age is identified as important to sickness absence, and most studies conclude that there is a positive correlation between the two. The basis for expecting a higher rate of sickness absence from the older part of the work force is that people will accumulate health problems during their (working) life and that they get tired and exhausted. Two decades ago, Tellnes (1989b) found that the duration of episodes of sickness absence increased with age: the mean days of sickness certification were about 50 days among elder workers (50+) and 30 days among young workers (20–49). This finding is also in accordance with more recent Norwegian studies and the annual statistics on sickness absence provided by Statistics Norway. In 2009, those in the age category 50+ had eight percent sickness absence compared to six percent among those aged 18–49 years (Statistics Norway 2010). It should be mentioned that some Swedish studies of age and sickness absence are less conclusive, indicating that age has little influence (Palmer 2004). The majority of former studies, however, tell us that we should expect a higher proportion of LTSA among the older workers compared to younger workers. We chose 49 years as the cut off-point between old and young workers (Tellnes 1989b; Statistics

Norway 2010). In the model, young workers (19–49) equal 0 (reference category), and older workers (50–67) equal 1.

There is also a growing literature on the effects of *family situation* and sickness absence. Some studies indicate that workers struggling to combine their work and family life have a higher risk of LTSA. Cohabitation and the presence of children may constitute higher demands at home (in particular, for women), and sickness absence could be an adverse outcome of this double work-home burden. Some research indicates weak relationships between the number of children and sickness absence, but it has also been found that being a single parent is associated with higher levels of sickness absence (Lidwall 2010). We expect that family conditions matter, and we differ between four household groups: single parents, couples with children, couples without children and single households. We expect single parents to have the highest level of LTSA and single households to have the lowest level of LTSA. The model uses single household as the reference category.

Some studies identify *education* as an important variable to sickness absence. Most of them either conclude that the risk of LTSA declines gradually with the number of years that people have studied (Labriola, Lund & Christensen 2007) or that people in the category 'low educational attainment' face a higher risk of LTSA than those with 'high educational attainment' (Lidwall 2010). We use the latter separation, and in our model, high educational attainment (bachelor level or higher) equals 0 (reference category), and low educational attainment (upper secondary or lower) equals 1.

A Danish status-of-knowledge report (Labriola, Lund & Christensen 2007) concludes that one of the factors that seem to influence the length of absence is whether a worker is employed in the *public or private sector*. According to this report, employees in the public sector have a higher risk of LTSA than their counterparts in the private sector. Contrary to this, Swedish studies report a tendency for people working for the municipalities (public sector) to end their sickness absence period faster than other workers (Palmer 2004). These opposite findings make it difficult to predict the relationship between sector and LTSA. In the regression model, private sector equals 0 (reference category), and public sector equals 1.

Psycho-social working conditions

How people perceive their psycho-social working conditions has proved to be important for sickness absence. There is extensive research in Norway and abroad on the relationship between the psycho-social conditions in working life and sickness absence. Various earlier studies have found that high demands and excessive work under pressure, the feeling of not being involved in major decisions concerning one's work situation, lack of opportunities to use skills and knowledge, and poor support from managers and colleagues are critical to sickness absence (Olsen & Mastekaasa 1997; Michi and Williams 2003; Ose et al. 2006). A lot of research on the psycho-social working conditions has been based on Karasek and Theorell's (1990) demand-control model. Little control and high demands expose people to a strain situation, and the lack of social support will accelerate the strain (Theorell 2004).

Our model tests the influence of psycho-social working conditions (PSWC) on LTSA by way of an index, ranging from a score of 5 (bad PSWC) to 25 (very good PSWC). The index on PSWC includes five variables. To what degree do you find that: i) the workload is satisfying, ii) you are appreciated by the manager and your colleagues, iii) the manager and colleagues give advice/offer to help with tasks that you find difficult, iv) your opinions are heard in decisions that involves your work situation, and v) you can use your skills and knowledge in the job. Empirical tests show a high level of internal consistency: Cronbach's α is 0.79, and all bivariate correlations are positive and medium strong (Pearson r varies from 0.3 to 0.53).

Social capital

In addition to the mainstream variables mentioned, we want to expand our understanding of LTSA. We suppose that the actual sickness absence is influenced by factors both inside and outside the work context, and the reported sickness absence will be a result of the informant's total situation. To account for social support outside the work place, we have included three indicators of the social capital that people report.

Social capital can be defined as resources available through membership in a network (Rønning & Starrin 2009). The notion of social capital applies to research areas such as social support, social trust, and social relations, and it relates to how well we are socially connected and integrated in the community

(Putnam 2000). We include three variables to capture whether or not networks and social capital are important for LTSA. The first variable is how often the respondent is visited by friends, family, and neighbours: once a month or more often equals 0 (reference category) and hardly ever equals 1. The second variable is participation or non-participation in nine common Norwegian organisations (union, industrial organization, political party, cultural group/organization, religious association/organization, environmental/leisure organization, sports association, humanitarian organization, and 'other' association/organization). In the model, active participation in one or more of these organisations equals 0 (reference category), and no active participation equals 1. The third variable concerns close friends: having one or more confidants equals 0 (reference category), and not having a confidant equals 1.

Life-style

In the current Norwegian debate about sickness absence, peoples' health has been an important topic. At the societal level, it is argued that peoples' health situation cannot explain a rise in sickness absence since the population is healthier than ever. At the individual level, it is shown that people's health situations matters for variations in sickness absence. It is well documented that life-style influence our health situation, and it is thus of interest to see if there is a connection between life-style and sickness absence.

The concept of life-style includes the sum of a person's living habits. Previous Scandinavian studies have documented that life-style risk factors (e.g. obesity, smoking) are associated with LTSA, but the causal pathways behind such associations are unclear (Allebeck & Mastekasa 2004; Lidwall 2010). A state-of-knowledge report on sickness absence comments on the (possible) effects of four life-style factors (Ose et al. 2006): smoking, use of alcohol, body-mass-index (BMI), and physical activity. Our data enables analysis on all these factors. The variable on smoking separates between those smoking each day (value 1) and those that do not (value 0). The variable on alcohol use separates between those who become intoxicated each week (value 1) and those that do not (value 0). The variable on BMI separates those belonging to the category obesity (BMI = 30+) (value 1) and those in categories underweight, normal weight, and overweight (BMI = -29) (value 0). Finally, on physical activity we separate between those who do not work out each week (value 1) and those who do work out each week (value 0).

Modelling

There is considerable research on the relationship between demographic variables and psycho-social conditions in working life and sickness absence, but less research on the correlations between life-style, social capital and sickness absence. By bringing all these factors into the same analysis, we hope that this chapter can bring new knowledge on factors of relevance to individual variations in LTSA.

The former section presented 15 variables expected to be relevant to self-reported LTSA. The influences of these dimensions on LTSA are investigated using a multivariate regression analysis. Regression analysis is an attempt to understand how a set of independent variables affects a particular dependent variable. In a multivariate model, the effect of each independent variable is controlled for by other variables. Logistic regression is suited when the dependent variable is dichotomous.

Causal modelling is fundamental to regression analysis. Causal modelling separates between exogenous variables (variables with no causal links leading to them from other variables in the model) and endogenous variables (variables with causal links leading to them from other variables in the model). A regression model assumes that independent variables are exogenous and that the dependent variable is endogenous. In practice, the classification of a particular variable may depend on the chosen causal model: the same variable may be exogenous in one model and endogenous in another model based on exactly the same set of variables.

In our model, LTSA is an endogenous variable. Gender and age are exogenous variables since they have no explicit causes within the model. Education, family situation and sector are both exogenous and endogenous: these variables could affect LTSA, but they could also be affected themselves by gender and age. Life-style, social capital and psycho-social working conditions are also both exogenous and endogenous: they could have an effect on LTSA, but they could themselves be affected by gender, age, education and sector. Furthermore, relations between life-style, social capital, psycho-social working conditions and sickness absence can go both ways: our model anticipates that LTSA is the dependent variable, but LTSA could be a relevant predictor if the dependent variable was assessment of either psycho-social working conditions or life-style or social capital. This illustrates the point above:

sometimes the classification of variables as either exogenous or endogenous depends on the chosen causal model.

Data

To discuss sickness absence, we use data on self-reported absence from a survey of level of living in Dovre and Lesja from 2009. All (approximately 2 000) households in Dovre and Lesja were visited by a representative from the data collectors, and one person in each household was invited to participate in the survey. The invited person was the member of the household between 16 and 79 years with the most recent birthday.

The net sample included 851 respondents, and that equals one fourth of the population in Dovre and Lesja in the relevant age category (16–79 years). The response rate to the survey was 43 percent and acceptable. The sample is not representative with regard to gender, age and household size: women are overrepresented (60 percent in the sample and 50 percent in the population); old people are overrepresented (mean age of 52 in the sample and 43 in the population); and households with one or two members are overrepresented (64 percent in the sample and 42 percent in the population). In the analysis on factors influencing sickness absence, we control for gender, age, and household type. The documentation report from the research project describes the research design in detail and gives a longer discussion about representativeness (Johansen & Rønning 2009).

The survey consisted of about 150 questions on different themes such as life-style, economy, health, social issues, and more. One large section was devoted to work, and approximately 560 employees ranging from 19 years of age to 67 years of age were invited to answer this section. Questions concerning sickness absence belonged to the section on work, and the survey included three questions about sickness absence:
- Question 1. Have you had doctor-certified and/or self-certified sickness absence during the last twelve months?
- Question 2. What was the main reason for your sickness absence?
- Question 3. For how long did you have sickness absence in the last twelve months?

The next section will present results on these questions, but we shall end this section with some comments on self-reported sickness absence and accuracy. The information given on questions about sickness absence relied entirely on the respondents' memory. Answers to questions about the past can be imperfect and thereby affect the validity of the results of the survey. The accuracy of recall depends on the time interval between the event and the time of its assessment: the longer the interval, the higher the probability of incorrect recalls. Previous research suggests that 20 percent of the critical details of a recognized event are irretrievable one year after its occurrence, while approximately half of critical details of a recognized event are irretrievable after five years (Hassan 2006). Our respondents were supposed to remember their sickness absence in the prior twelve months (one year). A related issue is response bias, which refers to instances when a respondent intentionally responds incorrectly to a question about their personal history. If this happened, then it would skew the survey results.

Response bias can be particularly problematic when you do interviews face-to-face or over the phone. Using such techniques to collect data, some respondents might be less likely to admit to sickness absence. There should be no interview effect in our data since respondents in Dovre and Lesja wrote down their answers on sickness absence in an anonymous survey. While we (probably) have no problem with response bias, recall bias is a completely different matter. The problem of recall is central to the most important variable: days of sickness absence in the last twelve months. 555 respondents answered whether they had sickness absence or not (Question 1), and 504 respondents answered with the number of days (Question 3). This tells us that one out of ten (50 respondents) could not remember the number of days they were absent in the last twelve months. Among those 504 that answered the question, it is difficult to tell about the accuracy of answers. We find it positive that most respondents (nine out of ten) have tried to remember the number of days in sickness absence, but we probably have a problem with accuracy, and that challenges the validity of results.

Descriptive analysis of sickness absence in Dovre and Lesja

The total sickness absence consists of absence certified by a doctor and self-certified absence. The Norwegian Labour and Welfare Administration are responsible for the official administrative registers (Sickness absence register and Employee register), and these registers include doctor-certified sickness absence and exclude self-certified sickness absence (Statistics Norway 2010). Therefore, to estimate the size of both self-certified absence and the total sickness absence we need to collect additional data. At the national level, Statistics Norway (2010) publishes results on self-certified sickness absence quarterly based on data reported by a sample of establishments. Due to sample size, these statistics are only presented by gender and type of industry and cannot be extracted to the municipality level. Thus, the self-certified sickness absence in Dovre and Lesja had not been measured before we did our survey on level of living in 2009. Our study of 555 employees shows that (question 1):

- 61 percent of the respondents had neither doctor-certified nor self-certified sickness absence in the prior twelve months
- 21 percent of the respondents had doctor-certified sickness absence
- 13 percent of the respondents had self-certified sickness absence
- five percent had both doctor-certified and self-certified sickness absence

These results tell us that approximately four out of ten respondents had sickness absence last year. Of those with sickness absence (39 percent of the respondents), the majority had doctor-certification (26 percent), and almost half had self-certified sickness absence (18 percent). At the national level, Statistics Norway (2010) estimates that 12–14 percent of the total sickness absence was self-certified, and 86–88 percent was doctor-certified in the past decade. In Dovre and Lesja, 87 percent of the total sickness absence was from respondents with doctor-certified sickness absence, four percent of the total absence was from respondents with self-certified sickness absence, and nine percent was from respondents with both doctor-certified absence and self-certified absence. We do not know the exact distribution of days amongst those with both doctor-certified and self-certified sickness absence, but it is likely that the major share is doctor-certified. Thus, it seems that Dovre and Lesja have a lower level of self-certified sickness absence compared to the national average.

The next issue was the causes for absence (Question 2). 31 percent of the respondents said that their absence was caused by 'pain in back, neck, knuckle, and muscles', eight percent answered that the main reason was mental problems, seven percent said their absence was due to either an injury or an accident, five percent claimed that they were certified sick due to heart illness, vascular illness, or cancer, and 49 percent referred to other causes. According to national statistics, musculoskeletal and mental problems are the most typical diagnoses in Norway: almost 40 percent of the doctor-certified absence is caused by musculoskeletal problems, and 18 percent is caused by mental problems. According to the respondents in Dovre and Lesja, 43 percent of their total absence (measured in days) was caused by pain in back, neck, knuckle, and muscles, 16 percent was caused by heart illness, vascular illness, or cancer, twelve percent was caused by psychic problems, five percent was caused by injury/accident, and 24 percent referred to other reasons.

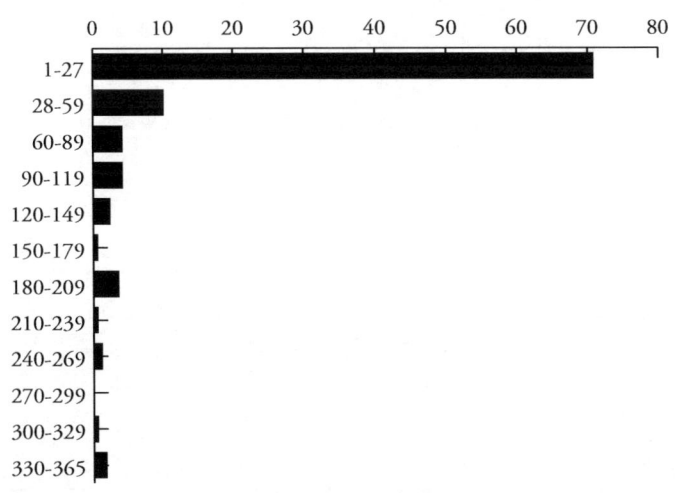

Figure 1: Distribution of days on sickness absence among those with sickness absence, percent. Source: Johansen & Rønning 2009.

The final query was about the number of days of sickness absence in the prior twelve months (question 3). Among those having sickness absence, the mean number of days on sickness absence is as high as 38. When we include those without sickness absence, the mean days of sickness absence drop to eleven. The mean becomes higher in skewed distributions with extreme values (such as 365 days on sickness absence, see fig. 1), and therefore the median is considered a better measure of the central tendency. The median divides the distribution of days on sickness absence in half, one with employees above the median and the other with employees below the median. The median among those with sickness absence is twelve days.

We are particularly interested in those with LTSA, here defined as at least 28 days within the last year. This group is shown in the grey area of figure 1.71 percent of all absentees (i.e. absent one to 365 days) were absent from one to 27 days, and 29 percent were absent from 28 to 365 days. Those with long-term sick absence (LTSA) account for 86 percent of the total sickness absence in Dovre and Lesja, and a mere 14 percent is accounted by the majority of 71 percent with short-term sickness absence (STSA). Of all workers responding to this question, approximately eight percent belong to the category with LTSA, 31 percent belong to the group with STSA, and 61 percent have no sickness absence.

Factors influencing long-term sickness absence

Section 2 presented 15 variables of relevance to long-term sickness absence (LTSA). This section presents the analysis of factors influencing LTSA.

Table 1: The factors influencing long-term sickness absence, unstandardized coefficients (B), p-value (p), standard error (SE) and odds ratio (Exp(B)).

Name of variable	B	p-value	SE	Exp(B)
Constant	-2.38	**	1.20	0.09
Woman	0.30		0.37	1.35
Older workers (50–67)	0.66		0.47	1.93
Couples without children	1.42	**	0.58	4.15
Single parents (0–17)	1.34		0.95	3.80
Couples with children (0–17)	1.03		0.66	2.79
Low educational attainment	0.46		0.43	1.58
Psycho-social working conditions	-0.12	**	0.05	0.88
Hardly ever visited by friends, family and neighbours	0.39		0.51	1.47
Not having a confidential friend	0.61		0.44	1.84
Daily smoking	0.85	**	0.39	2.35
Obesity (BMI)	0.51		0.50	1.67
Nagelkerke R^2	0.14			

*** Significant at 0.01, ** Significant at 0.05, * Significant at 0.1.
Reference categories: Man; younger workers (19–49); single household; high educational attainment; monthly visits by friends, family & neighbours; having a confidential friend; not smoking on a daily basis; not obesity

The best-fit model includes eleven variables, and that means that four of the variables presented in section 2 are excluded due to lack of explanatory power. These variables are sector, participating in organisations, intoxication, and physical training. The original model is found in the appendix (table 2). Table 1 presents the best-fit model, and it includes these variables: women, older workers, couples without children, single parents, couples with children, low educational attainment, psycho-social working conditions, hardly ever visited by friends/family/neighbours, not having a confidential friend, daily smoking, and obesity.

The first column gives the name of the variables included in the analysis. The second column shows the unstandardized Coefficient (B): the average increase in the dependent variable with one measurement increase in X (the independent variable) when other independent variables are held constant. The third column presents the p-value: the probability that X and Y are not related. The fourth column presents the standard of errors (SE): small numbers indicate little sample-to-sample variation, and larger numbers indicate the opposite (Hamilton 1992). The fifth column presents odds ratios: the probability of the outcome event occurring divided by the probability of the event not occurring. We will focus our comments on p-values and the odds ratio, but the first thing to comment on is Nagelkerke R^2.

In linear regression analysis, R^2 is a measure of goodness-of-fit. Corresponding, logistic regression models enables calculations of R^2-like measures, and the most reported of the pseudo R^2-estimates is Nagelkerke R^2. Nagelkerke R^2 ranges from 0 to 1, and higher values indicate better model fit. Table 1 includes eleven variables and Nagelkerke R^2 is 0.14. This is an acceptable result, even if there is still a lot of variance in LTSA left unexplained. Our interpretation is that the model includes some important variables and some less relevant variables.

While Nagelkerke R^2 assesses the strength of the whole model, p-values give an indication of the impact of each single variable. A null hypothesis (H_0) is the prediction that an observed difference is due to chance alone and not due to a systematic cause, and p-values are measures of how probable that data was, assuming the null hypothesis is true. If the data appears very improbable (usually defined as a type of data that should be observed less than five percent of the time, $p< 0.05$), then the conclusion is that the null hypothesis is false and effects are statistical significant. Through this test, we find statistical significant effects for these variables: couples without children, psycho-social working conditions and daily smoking. The remaining variables in the model are non-significant, but some of them are close to the 0.1-level (p<0.10).

Odds ratios (last column) present an additional way of interpreting results. The 'odds' of an event is calculated by the probability of the outcome event occurring divided by the probability of the event not occurring. When the odds ratio is close to 1, we do not have any particular effect; the higher it is over 1, the stronger the positive effect, and the closer it is to 0, the stronger the negative effect.

We begin with a look at the impact for the variables representing our particular areas of interest: life-style and social capital. On life-style, we find that the model estimates that daily smokers are 2.3 times more likely to have LTSA compared to non-smokers and less frequent smokers. It also calculates that people in the obesity category are 1.7 times more likely to have LTSA than those with a lower BMI. On the matter of social capital, we find that those without a confidant are 1.8 times more likely to have long-term absence compared to those with one or more close friends. And the risk of LTSA is 1.5 times higher for people hardly ever visited by friends, family, and neighbours than those with regular or monthly visits.

Odds ratios are also calculated for the other variables in the model. It is not a surprise that psycho-social working conditions are important: the risk of LTSA rises eleven percent for each point decrease in the assessment of psycho-social working conditions. Family situation is also very important: couples without children and single parents are about four times more likely to have LTSA than single people, and the odds for couples with children is 2.8 times greater than for single people. Furthermore, the model estimates that older workers (50–67 years) are 1.9 times more likely to have LTSA than younger workers (19–49 years). It is also estimated that the risk of LTSA is 1.6 times higher for people with low educational attainment than those with high educational attainment. Finally, women are 1.4 times more likely to have LTSA than men.

Final comments

Sickness absence is a complex phenomenon, and different perspectives are useful when explaining its size and variation. The most applied models of factors of relevance to sickness absence seem to include three elements: individual factors, aspects of work, and aspects of society (Lidwall 2010). Using data from a study in Dovre and Lesja with more than 500 employees, this chapter has discussed the influences of individual factors and psycho-social work aspects to variations in long-term sickness absence (LTSA).

Even if we do not account for all variables of relevance to sickness absence, the main strength of our study is the possibility to analyze an array of variables at the same time. Another positive side to our study is that we account for both doctor-certified and self-certified sickness absence. One vital limit to our study is that we probably have problem with recall bias: some respondents found it hard to remember the exact number of days they were absent in the prior twelve months. Another limit is that we lack the possibility to trace causal relationships. Here we need more research to follow up.

Our analysis showed that four variables expected to matter did not influence sickness absence. First, working in the private sector does not seem to imply a lower rate of sickness absence compared to working in the public sector. Nor did we find our expected correlations for the use of alcohol, physical training, or membership in organizations. The latter variable was one of three indicators of social capital, and the two former were indicators of life-style.

The other variables in our model proved various degrees of influence on LTSA. First, substantial attention has been paid to psycho-social conditions in the workplace. Associations between sickness absence and the psycho-social work environment are theoretically illustrated by the demand-control model (Karasek & Theorell 1990), and the correlation between our index of psycho-social working conditions and LTSA was strong in our data. This is an important finding. Studies on the psycho-social working conditions have often been conducted in one or few organizations (Gamperiene et al. 2007), which restrict the possibilities for generalization. Our data is better suited for generalizations: we were able to test the effect of psycho-social working conditions on the whole population of employees in two municipalities.

Secondly, the family situation proved important. Former studies have indicated that family conditions like cohabitation and the presence of children might add to the workload and stress experienced by employees (Lidwall 2010). The importance of family was strong in our data: single people were markedly less likely to have LTSA than couples without children, single parents, and couples with children. Third, we also found that education, gender, and age mattered. In particular, LTSA was more frequent for the elderly part of the working population than for the younger.

Of most interest are perhaps the final sets of variables added in our study: life-style and social capital. In our model, life-style was measured by smoking and BMI. Life-style factors such as daily smoking and obesity are usually part of more complex life-style patterns associated with increased health risks. Since life-style influences health, and there is a strong association between health and sickness absence, we also expect there to be a relation between life-style and LTSA. Our findings indicate that it may be useful to conduct more research on the correlations between life-style indicators and sickness absence. In particular, it seems that daily smoking matters to LTSA. For the employers, our preliminary findings will provide support for a focus on life-style and more health promotion.

Social capital relates to how well we are socially connected and integrated in the community (Putnam 1990). In our model, we find that respondents hardly ever visited by friends, family, and neighbours and without a friend to confide in are overrepresented with LTSA. With this, our findings indicate that the 'total situation' matters: both social supports inside and outside the work-place is important to LTSA. Further research is needed to understand the relations between external and internal support. An interesting follow-up investigation could be to see whether external and internal support can compensate for each other, or whether they represent different types of social support such that we need both.

References

Allebeck, Peter & Arne Mastekaasa 2004. 'Risk factors for sick leave – general studies'. *Scandinavian Journal of Public Health*, no. 63, 49–108

Gamperiene, Migle, Asbjørn Grimsmo & Bjørg Aase Sørensen 2007. *Programmet FARVE Kunnskapsstatus. Tema 1: Sykefravær.* Oslo, Work Research Institute (WRI working paper 1/2007)

Hamilton, Lawrence 1992. *Regression with graphics: A second course in applied statistics.* California, Wadsworth Inc

Hassan, Eman 2006. 'Recall Bias can be a Threat to Retrospective and Prospective Research Designs', *Internet Journal of Epidemiology* no. 2. http://www.ispub.com/ostia/index.php?xmlFilePath=journals/ije/vol3n2/bias.xml#h1–3

Hensing, Gunnel 2009. 'The measurements of sickness absence – a theoretical perspective'. *Norsk Epidemiologi* no. 2, 147–151

Hogstedt, Christer et al. eds. 2004. *Den höga sjukfråvaron – sanning och konsekvens*. Stockholm, Swedish National Institute of Public Health

Johansen, Vegard & Rolf Rønning 2009. *Levekår i Oppland: fordelinger for Dovre og Lesja*. Lillehammer, Eastern Norway Research Institute (ENRI working paper 07/2009)

Karasek, Robert & Tores Theorell 1990. *Healthy work: Stress, productivity, and the reconstruction of working life*. New York, Basic books

Labriola, Merete, Thomas Lund & Karl-Bang Christensen 2007. *Resultater av sygefraværsforskning 2003–2007*. København, National Research Centre for the Working Environment

Lidwall, Ulrik 2010. *Long-term sickness absence: aspects of society, work and family*. Stockholm, Karolinska Institutet

Mykletun, Arnstein et al. 2009. *Tiltak for reduksjon i sykefravær: Aktiviserings- og nærværsreform*. Oslo, Ministry of Labour

Olsen, Karen & Arne Mastekaasa 1997. *Forskning om sykefravær – en oppsummering og vurdering av perioden 1980–96*. Oslo, Institute for Social Research (ISR-rapport 3)

Ose, Solveig et al. 2006. *Sykefravær. Kunnskapsstatus og problemstillinger*. Trondheim, SINTEF (SINTEF report no. A325)

Palmer, Edward 2004. 'Sjukskrivningen i Sverige - inledande översikt'. Hogstedt, Christer et al. eds.: *Den höga sjukfråvaron – sanning och konsekvens*, 27–81

Putnam, Robert 2000. *Bowling alone*. New York, Simon & Schuster

Rønning, Rolf & Bengt Starrin eds. 2009. *Sosial kapital i et velferdsperspektiv*. Oslo, Gyldendal akademisk

Statistics Norway 2010. *Working conditions, sickness absenteeism*. http://www.ssb.no/english/subjects/06/02/

Tellnes, Gunnar 1989. 'Sickness certification in general practice: a review', *Family Practice* no. 1, 58–65.

Theorell, Tores 2004. 'Stressmekanismer och sjukskriving'. Hogstedt, Christer et al. eds.: *Den höga sjukfråvaron – sanning och konsekvens*, 255–79

Appendix

Table 2: Original model - the factors influencing long-term absence.

Variables	B	p-value	SE	Exp(B)
Constant	-2.37	*	1.32	0.09
Woman	0.22		0.40	1.25
Older workers (50–67)	0.60		0.48	1.82
Couples without children	1.43	**	0.60	4.16
Single parents	1.48		0.98	4.38
Couples with children	0.99		0.68	2.68
Low educational attainment	0.51		0.45	1.67
Public sector	0.01		0.40	1.01
Psycho-social working conditions	-0.11	**	0.05	0.89
Hardly ever visited by friends, family and neighbours	0.31		0.57	1.37
Non-active participation in organisations	-.362		0.39	0.70
Not having a confidential friend	0.64		0.48	1.90
Daily smoking	0.93	**	0.41	2.52
Weekly intoxicated by alcohol	0.38		0.90	1.46
Obesity (BMI)	0.57		0.53	1.77
Not working out each week	0.07		0.40	1.07
Nagelkerke R^2	0.14			

*** Significant at 0.01, ** Significant at 0.05, * Significant at 0.1.
Reference categories: Man; younger workers (19–49); single household; high educational attainment; private sector; monthly visits by friends, family and neighbours; active participation in one or more organisations; having a confidential friend; not smoking on a daily basis; not weekly intoxicated by alcohol; not obesity; working out each week

Authors

Kari Batt-Rawden is a sociologist with a salutogenetic approach to health and illness issues. She is working as a researcher at the Eastern Norway Research Institute (Østlandsforskning) in Lillehammer. Her PhD research on music and health promotion won a Strong Commendation from the Royal Society for Public Health. Batt-Rawden also belongs to the Sociology of the Arts group at Exeter University.
 Email: kbr@ostforsk.no

Lena Ede has a bachelor degree in social science and is a PhD student in the Department of Social Studies at Karlstad University, in Sweden. She is also working as a research assistant at Eastern Norway Research Institute (Østlandsforskning). Her research interests concern work environment, care work, and long-term sickness absence.
 E-mail: lena.ede@kau.se

Lars-Gunnar Engström has a PhD in Public Health Sciences and is a Senior Lecturer at the Department of Social Work at Karlstad University in Sweden. His major research interests concern public health, sickness absence, and gender.
 E-mail: lars-gunnar.engstrom@kau.se

Ulla-Britt Eriksson has a PhD in Public Health Sciences, is a Senior Lecturer at the Department of Health and Environmental Sciences at Karlstad University in Sweden and is a Senior Researcher at Eastern Norway Research

Institute. Her major research interests concern public health, social relations, and sickness absence.

E-mail: ulla-britt.eriksson@kau.se

Bjørn Hofmann is a Professor at the University College of Gjøvik, an Adjunct Professor at the Section for medical ethics at the University of Oslo, and a researcher at the Norwegian Knowledge Center for the Health Services. His main research interests are in philosophy of science and medicine, technology assessment, and bioethics.

E-mail: bjoern.hofmann@hig.no

Staffan Janson, MD, PhD, is a Senior Pediatrician, a Professor of Public Health at Karlstad University, and a Professor of Social Pediatrics at Örebro University in Sweden. He is also attached to Eastern Norway Research Institute. His major interest is in social and environmental determinants of child and adult health.

E-mail: staffan.janson@kau.se

Vegard Johansen received a PhD in Political Science from the Norwegian University of Science and Technology. He is Senior Researcher at the Eastern Norway Research Institute and holds seminars in quantitative methods. His main research interests are entrepreneurship education, children's welfare, and European welfare policies.

E-mail: vj@ostforsk.no

Halvor Nordby graduated with a D.Phil in philosophy from the University of Oxford in 2001. He is currently a Professor at Lillehammer University College in the Faculty of Health and Social Work, and he is also working at the University of Oslo in the Faculty of Medicine. His main areas of research include communication, health care, and social work.

E-mail: halvor.nordby@hil.no

Rolf Rønning is a Professor at Lillehammer University College and is affiliated with the Eastern Norway Research Institute. He has worked and published on topics within social policy for more than thirty years. His main areas of interest have been elderly care and the situation for social benefit recipients. He is currently engaged with innovation in welfare services.

E-mail: rolf.ronning@hil.no

Tuva Schanke received a Masters of Science in Education from the Norwegian University of Science and Technology. Her specialization was in Counselling, a programme both theoretically and practically directed towards educational-psychological counseling. She works as a Researcher at the Eastern Norway Research Institute. Her research interests include employment research, career counselling, and entrepreneurship education.

E-mail: tsc@ostforsk.no

Liv Johanne Solheim has been an Associate Professor in the Faculty of Health and Social Work at Lillehammer University College since 1995 and is a former senior researcher at Eastern Norway Research Institute. Her major research interests include social policy, activation, marginalization processes, and inclusive working life.

Email: liv.solheim@hil.no

Bengt Starrin has a PhD in Sociology and is a Professor of Social Work at the Department of Social Studies at Karlstad University, Sweden, an Adjunct Professor of Social Policy at Faculty of Health and Social Studies, Lillehammer University College and a senior researcher at Eastern Norway Researc Institute. His major research interests concern the sociology of emotions, public health, social policy, and welfare.

Email: Bengt.Starrin@kau.se

Gunnar Tellnes, MD, received a PhD from the University of Oslo (UiO) in 1990 for his work on 'Doctors' sickness certification practice'. Since 1991, he has been a Professor in Social Insurance Medicine (trygdemedisin) at UiO and a specialist in Community Medicine. Today, he is parttime Senior Consultant at Norwegian Labour and Welfare (NAV Buskerud).

Email: gunnar.tellnes@medisin.uio.no